'The universe is a tree eternally existing. Its root aloft, its branches spread below. The pure root of the tree is Brahman the immortal, in whom the three worlds have their being, whom none can transcend, who is verily the Self.'

Katha Upanishad, VI, I

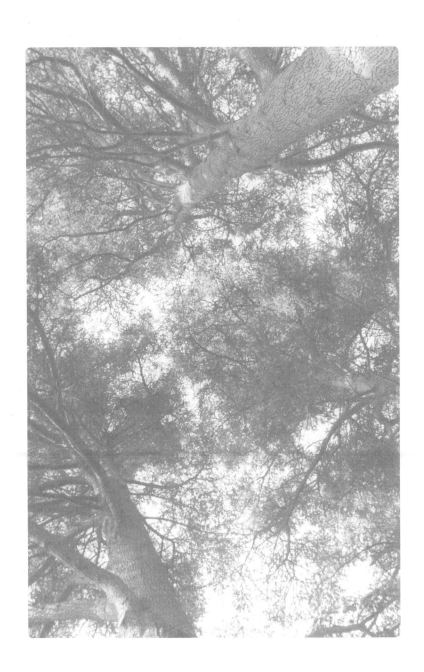

TREE
YOGA

A WORKBOOK

*Strengthen Your Personal
Yoga Practice Through the
Living Wisdom of Trees*

Satya Singh
Fred Hageneder

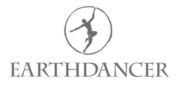

EARTHDANCER

A FINDHORN PRESS IMPRINT

1 2 3 4 5 6 7 21 20 19 18 17 16 15 14 13 12 11 10 09 08 07

Tree Yoga
Satya Singh & Fred Hageneder

This English edition © 2007 Earthdancer GmbH
English translation © 2007 Sam Bloomfield

Originally published in German as *Baum-Yoga*

World copyright © 2006 Neue Erde GmbH, Saarbruecken, Germany
Original German text copyright © 2005 Satya Singh & Fred Hageneder

Cover design: Dragon Design UK
Cover photography: Satya Singh

Editing & proofreading: Claudine Bloomfield
Book design and typography: Dragon Design UK
Typeset in Berkeley

Printed and bound in China

ISBN 978-1-84409-119-5

Published by Earthdancer GmbH, an imprint of:
Findhorn Press, 305a The Park, Findhorn, Forres IV36 3TE, Great Britain
www.earthdancer.co.uk – www.findhornpress.com

Contents

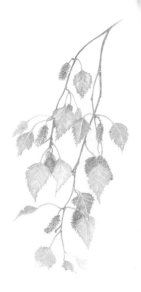

'You can learn from a tree to stand in ecstasy.'

Yogi Bhajan

Foreword

Each and every tree has a unique way of being that each of us can recognise. The birch has the light playfulness of a child; the radiant colours of the rowan tree can inspire us, while the Yew exudes an utterly sublime sense of stillness. Intensively practice Yogi Bhajan's Kundalini Yoga, and you too can recognise these energies. Doing these exercises is just like drawing the energies of the trees into ourselves.

The idea of this book is to bring together the extraordinary worlds of yoga and trees. It was no coincidence that the Buddha became enlightened while sitting under a bodhi tree. At that time in India the bodhi was already worshipped for its superior wisdom. Nor was it a coincidence that Yogi Bhajan was brought to a bodhi tree by his master, Sant Hazara Singh, to spend three days and nights living in its crown.

Yoga that is practiced under or near a tree is made more powerful by the aura of that tree. Practice yoga under an oak, for example, and absorb the power and determination that it radiates, thus becoming more reliable and steadfast yourself. Or go under a beech tree to elevate your focus and clarity of mind. And more than this, every tree that you encounter is an invitation to your heart to return the love and blessings that this wonderful being is giving you.

This book contains an introduction to the spiritual significance of trees. You will find twelve species: eleven European trees, and the pipal or bodhi tree from India. Each species is accompanied by meditations and exercises. The meditations come from the brimming cup of techniques that Yogi Bhajan taught to his students from 1969 onwards, when he came to the West from India. The symbiosis of European trees with ancient Indian techniques is obviously a modern event. But it is also a synergy that is the result of careful selection, years of experience, and pure inspiration.

In choosing the exercises to share with you here, we have given a particular focus to the standing poses. This choice was inspired by the following quote by Yogi Bhajan:

'You can learn from a tree to stand in ecstasy.'

The standing poses are also really practical because mother nature's floor tends to be a bit damp at times.

These exercises are not *kriyas* or sets as traditionally practiced in Kundalini Yoga. Instead the different series' of exercises are designed to bring us into harmony with the energies of a particular species of tree.

We dedicate this book to Yogi Bhajan with our greatest thanks for the many fruit-bearing branches that have grown from the powerful roots of his teachings. His having left this world on the 6th of October 2004 has unfortunately prevented us from showing him this book, yet we believe that he would have very much enjoyed it because he so loved trees.

June 2007
Satya Singh, Hamburg, Germany
Fred Hageneder, Stroud, England

Part I

Veda

'There is a banyan tree which has its roots upward and its branches down, and whose leaves are the Vedic hymns. One who knows this tree is the knower of the Vedas.'

Bhagavad-Gita, XVl, 1

Beginnings

At the beginning, in the endless depths of nothingness, there appeared one tiny point. This, the navel of the world, already contained within itself the whole of the universe, and was soon to unfurl itself like a sapling from a seed. While the *physical* cosmos manifests itself predominantly in spherical forms and movements, as planets, stars, orbits and spiralling galaxies; the *spiritual* aspect of the universe unfolds in the form of a tree.

Everything in existence is a part of the organic unity of this, the World Tree. In the material world it looks like one thing is separate from another, but in reality all things are not just interconnected, but are *as one*. The ever present and all-encompassing spirit doesn't just belong to human beings. It is not born of the partial mind of humans, but is the immortal root of all being. We know it as the quality we call *love*.

All beings in creation are holy, as each are a part of the *one* organism, the World Tree; the Tree of Life. Human beings are particularly valuable because of the capacity of free will, which can make them into nature's tools, capable of producing love and empathy in the physical world. Animals are particularly valuable because they are the realisation of the creative diversity of soul (Anima – *animals*). Plants and especially trees are so valuable because they embody, in its purest form, the very flesh of the immortal Tree of Life. Part of their quality, then, is the bringing of this healing energy into the physical world.

The foundations of the above thoughts are tens of thousands of years old, forming part of the world picture of our Neolithic forebears. Archaeological finds depicting the World Tree date back in

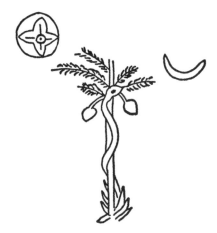

Fig. 1. Neolithic symbol of the World Tree with snake (discovered in Elam, Persia)

excess of 40,000 years. Throughout this age and beyond, groups of humans wandered the face of the planet, populating landscapes hitherto unknown to them, integrating with indigenous peoples and forming new groups that then travelled on. These groups took the ancient symbol of the World Tree with them; and as the different cultures of humanity were formed, the symbol of the World Tree took on different forms. Yet while the attributes, holy names and rituals changed, the essence remained the same. So, when it comes to celebrating this sacred tree and understanding its deeper meaning we discover today a remarkable agreement, between the most geographically disparate cultures, agreement that has spanned millennia.

The most important characteristics in the cosmology of the Tree of Life are:

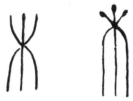

Fig. 2. On the right you can see the pre-dynastic hieroglyph of ancient Egypt (circa 3000 BC) for birth, which is derived from the hieroglyph on the left that means tree.

- The Tree of Life is the source of all things. Every living thing comes from this being who holds both the masculine and feminine polarities within itself. Its seeds contain the form of everything about to become life. We could say that this being is the great mother who nourishes all, and contains the means for the final healing of all suffering.

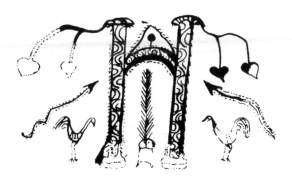

Fig. 3a. Two metaphysical guards usually protect the Tree of Life, in this case – a motif from the Celtic La Tène – two snakes and two birds.

About 2,600 years ago, the Persian high priest Zarathustra had the following to say about the World Tree: 'Honour to Haoma. He is good, well and truly born, the giver of welfare and health, victorious and of golden hue; his branches bow down that one may enjoy them. To the soul he is the way to heaven.'

● According to the mythology of the ancient world, the Tree of Life stands in a paradisiacal garden as the symbol of creation in the place of enlightenment. A magical being protects it, usually a snake, dragon or cherubim. The guardians are often a pair, which refers to the duality of human consciousness, where we find the left brain as logical and the right brain as intuitive. This suggests that we have to conquer duality before becoming as one with the World Tree that is the soul of the world.

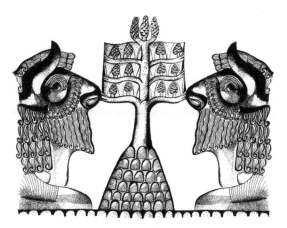

Fig. 3b. In the ancient Orient, the guardians of the World Tree were usually two cherubim, as you can see in this relief on a pre-Persian stone dish from Susa (circa 2300 BC).

● The Tree of Life is the fundamental ground of the eternal, invisible universe, which lies behind the world of appearances that we think of as reality. The essence of this tree is spirit, and as such the tree of knowledge is our path to true understanding, spiritual growth and enlightenment. The most widely known spiritual example for this kind of human development is the Buddha (see also the bodhi tree p. 172).

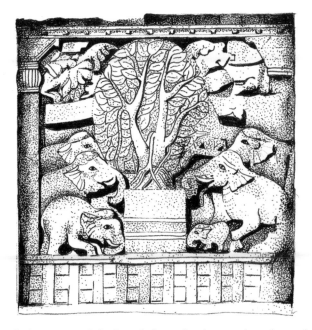

Fig. 4. The human search for knowledge under the sacred tree has endured since the beginning of time. Originally the Buddha was symbolised by an empty throne at the foot of the bodhi tree (the Tree of Enlightenment). He conquered the boundaries of body and ego, becoming one with the cosmic tree. This image of the Stupa of Bharhut shows the invisible Buddha being paid homage to by elephants.

- The essence of the Tree of Life is a substance that can give health and even immortality. Some myths depict this substance as fruit: for the Greeks, apples from the tree of Hesperides; or in Germanic myth, the apples of Iduna. Other traditions have this substance as the tree's sap (*homa* in ancient Persia, *soma* in India). This nectar of the gods also delivers omniscience. In Celtic and Germanic myth, this nectar is boiled in a magical cauldron owned by the gods themselves.

Grove and Temple

Humans have long chosen mighty trees or powerful groves to celebrate the fruitfulness and generosity of nature. These kinds of places were chosen as shrines by most early cultures. Of course people also needed timber for building, burning, tools and furniture, and because of this need parts of the ancient forests were regularly harvested and coppiced as far back as pre-historic times.* But where they took, people also gave in return. Their offerings took the form of prayers and blessings, and all sorts of sacrificial offerings like flowers, fruits, food in general, water, milk, beer, wine and tobacco. Other gifts included valuable objects made from wood or metal. Yet more important than the nutritional or physical sacrifice was, and is still today, the consciousness behind it: the love, the offering, and the sense of profound gratitude.

Throughout the evolution of humanity, sacred groves and trees (along with springs, caves, mountaintops and fires) have been the places to engage in religious activity. This is true of the Celtic, Germanic, Slavic, Baltic, and Finno -Ugric peoples of Europe and Asia; and also true of the Romans, Greeks, Oriental peoples, ancient Chinese, Japanese; and many African, Australian and American indigenous peoples.

Very early on in the history of global tree worship we find altars appearing under holy trees; canopies followed, then roofs,

---

* Coppicing is a type of forestry where trees are cut almost to the ground every 4 to 10 years. Species such as hazelnut, ash and willow grow faster when coppiced, and can live much longer than if left to grow naturally.

and finally whole temples. Most holy places, and practically all temple gardens and groves, were carefully guarded through the ages. Yet, gradually, as a change in the religious impulse of human beings led them to explore their inner dimensions, the groves and trees next to the temples became largely forgotten. Only the exquisite complex of the Acropolis in Athens kept the goddess Athena's sacred olive tree at its heart.

Christian history, too, was influenced by the sacredness of trees. Early Christian holy men usually chose lives of poverty and renunciation, living in simple stone huts or hollow trees. In Ireland they often chose ancient yews. Once there, they usually preached under the canopy of such trees. Some of these tree dwellings later developed into large monasteries and educational centres.

Tree and Human

A brief scientific look at trees can show us why people from all over the world decided to turn them into temples, searching out their presence for healing, and expanding consciousness.

It was in 1925 that the electrical current of a tree (a maple) was first measured and documented. An extended research project undertaken by Yale University in 1943–1966 established without a shadow of doubt that trees exist within a bioelectrical field.

The charge within the electrical field of trees follows a rhythmical pattern. The voltage is at its lowest in the early morning and at its highest at noon. During the year in the northern hemisphere, a tree's lowest voltage is found in April and its highest in September. The bioelectrical fields of trees react to very subtle changes in light, atmospheric charge and the earth's magnetic field. They mirror the phases of the moon, and also the eleven-year cycle of solar flare activity. Every species of tree has developed its own particular characteristics based on these earthly and cosmic rhythms. For example, the electromagnetic activity of a birch is about double that of a pine with the same trunk thickness. In this sense, oaks are the most energised trees we have around us. But there is more to this than trees just reacting to environmental conditions. Plants have the ability to influence their own electrical activity. It has been proved that they can initiate their own electrical processes.

If we look at the role of electricity, we can see that it plays a very central role in the metabolism of all biological life forms. Plant cells are only able to absorb nutrients because the nutrients carry the opposite electrical charge to the plant cells. Photosynthesis is also a largely bioelectrical process. If you want to know in detail about the themes raised in this introduction, take a look at Fred's book *The Spirit of Trees*.

Trees don't only partake in their own bioelectrical processes, which mainly take place in the living layer of cells beneath the bark and in the leaves; they also constantly feed the positive charge of the ionosphere into the earth's crust, which is negatively charged. One of the simple laws of physics tells us that a live conductor of electricity gives off its own electromagnetic field. The dispute over whether trees possess their own aura can now be laid to rest.

Because the electrically active layers can be found just under the bark, hugging trees has a deeply vitalising effect on us. The same is true for sitting with your back resting on a tree. There is no doubt that doing this leads to reciprocal stimulation for both human and tree. Doing this means that the flow of energy going through the tree can directly interact with the spine and energetic processes of the human brain.

If you sensitise yourself to this delicate current you will even discover that just being within the energy field of the tree, so anywhere under the whole of the crown, is just as powerful as being right next to the trunk.

More remarkable yet is the fact that trees are receivers and amplifiers of cosmic rays. The buds of trees, in their many different forms and sizes, react to different frequencies of energy waves as specially calibrated antenna. We see this story repeated at the microscopic level throughout the proportions and structures of the cell organs. This organisational coherence continues to the DNA strands themselves, which are perfectly tuned to the frequency of sunlight.

In the last few years, biophysics has discovered the existence of bio-photons. Rays of light, electromagnetic waves, warmth and sound can all electrically stimulate molecules in cells, allowing these previously captured bio-photons to stream out from the cells. All organic tissue sends out bio-photons. According to physics, the bio-photon field of a healthy organism shows a very high degree of order, and is capable of stimulating other living structures and passing information to them to further their own coherence. Experiments have shown that bio-photon radiation can travel through thousands of cells with very little energy loss. Furthermore, individual cells can respond to this information if they find it useful. The whole of the bio-photon field directs the course that an organism takes throughout its life. Signals such as an immune response or the generation of tissue can be sent to every part of the body at the speed of light. Communication in living organisms therefore actually happens far quicker than just through the chemical hormonal system.

The DNA, as well as working together with a whole hierarchy of light-active molecules, is both main store and transmitter of bio-photon radiation. It is also capable of absorbing a beam of light with one of its strands and then later sending out this light once more from a different strand, at the same time altering its frequency.

Our bodies do this, as do trees' bodies. The many aspects of the energy field of a tree, including the electromagnetic, are invisible to the human eye. Yet, if you find yourself under the crown of a large tree you are actually in the midst of an awesome fireworks show, which both envelops you and penetrates right through you.

The Indo-European Connection

Because tree yoga brings together Vedic and Druidic impulses, it seems like a good idea to take a short look at how two apparently so different cultural groups relate to each other.

History tells us that at some point during the second millennia BC, patriarchal, horse-riding tribes from the Middle East reached Europe and blended with more matriarchal, indigenous, agricultural communities. The following centuries saw the results of this as the development of Celtic, Germanic, Slavic and Baltic cultures. During the same period, other groups originating from the same area wandered into what is now Persia, and beyond into the Indian subcontinent. This explains the vast spread, from Ireland to India, of Indo-European languages.

But it isn't just in the language of Indo-European peoples that we see many aspects in common, but also in culture, and especially religion. An example of this, as already mentioned, is the Tree of Life, which was uniformly known to and worshipped by both invaders and indigenous peoples. We know this because it had been worshipped since the late Middle Stone Age.

Countless other aspects of world-view and religious practice show us interesting parallels. This becomes particularly clear if we compare Celtic Druids with Vedic Brahmans, for example:

● The cosmology of both religious cultures is very similar. According to both, the universe has four levels: the kingdom of the eternal spirit, an astral world where both ghosts and demigods exist, an 'otherworld' of mostly ethereal nature, and the physical world.

- The myths of both personify deities of spirit and primeval nature energies. Celtic deities are known as *deuos* meaning 'the shining', while the Vedic deities are known as *devas*, which means 'the shining ones'.

- Both cultures hold the view that the immortal soul continues to exist after death in the astral planes until such a time as the person or animal takes on physical form again.

- In both Celtic and Vedic traditions, the whole universe goes through cycles of life and death.

- In the past, both Druids and Brahmans received their sacred teachings orally and then transmitted them from memory. Writing them down was forbidden. Both *professions* included prophets, judges, royal advisors and leaders of rituals, as well as healers and astrologers.

- Just like Brahmans, Druids practice conscious breathing, posture and meditation techniques aimed at their spiritual development.

- In a very disciplined manner, both had to study natural sciences, law, ritual, mathematics, and astronomy. Brahmans also had to learn astrology, studying for 12 years in all, while Druids studied over a twenty-year period.

- The storytellers and songsters (bards) of both traditions learnt very long poems by heart. The poetic meter consisted of lines with the same number of syllabi, with a three-part cadence at the end.

• Both religions praised the magical power of words and the importance of speaking the truth, and placed great value on articulacy.

• Both cultures had female seers, and priestesses were the preferred choice for rituals dedicated to goddesses.

• Celtic society was made up of three groups; Druids and bards, a warrior aristocracy, and producers (including the trades). It was possible to change from one group to the other. Vedic society was made up of four castes: priests, warriors, traders, and producers. It is suggested in the Veda that movement between the castes was possible; but in time their social structure became more rigid, rather inhibiting the organic evolution of the individual.

It is the last point, at least from a modern perspective, that highlights the biggest difference between the two cultures. Unlike Brahmans under the frozen Indian caste system, Druids were not *born* as such; anyone could put themselves forward for a Druidic education. The equality of women also persisted in Celtic society until the Roman conquest, while it was lost early on in the development of the Vedic culture.

The social and religious impulses of Guru Nanak in sixteenth century India arrived to bring things back into balance. With his teachings and the establishment of Sikh Dharma, he began a process of bringing the democratic principles of a level playing field and female equality back to Indian society.

Kundalini Yoga

'Kundalini Mata Shakti, Mata Shakti Namo Namo'
(*Kundalini, mother energy, mother energy I call you, I call you*)

Different cultures have handed down the traditional wisdom of there being a World Tree *inside* the human body. Ancient Egyptian sources, as well as the mystical writings of Jewish rabbis, talk of the importance of the spine as being the *root* containing an awesome amount of life force and consciousness. A complete teaching for the care of this, our 'own' Tree of Life, comparable to the Taoist alchemical tradition of ancient China, has been gifted to us by Yogi Bhajan as Kundalini Yoga.

The word *kundal* means 'spiral', 'coil', or 'to be coiled up'. The word *Kundalini* describes the highest possible human energy state. It refers to a god-like energy, which has been psychically seen to lie curled three times around the lowest energy centre in

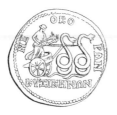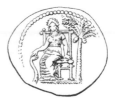

Fig. 5. A well known picture from antiquity shows deities, in particular feminine ones, served and befriended by snake energy. Three Greek coins from the fifth to the first century BC: on the left you can see the goddess Demeter riding her snake-drawn carriage; in the centre, goddess of the underworld, Persephone; and on the right an unknown goddess from Crete, under a date palm.

each one of us, like a serpent, or – as Yogi Bhajan described it – like the curling lock of the beloved. This energy centre is called the root *chakra*. The word *chakra* means 'wheel' and 'energy centre'.

If this energy begins to move and spontaneously starts to ascend without preparation, the transformations that can result can be hard to cope with. But if we allow this energy to grow like a tree, by, for example, practicing Kundalini Yoga, it empowers the human soul to consciously and increasingly manifest into our everyday lives.

The classical description of when and how Kundalini energy is awakened is full of tree symbolism. This begins with the two basic energies of the human being: *prana* and *apana*.

As a tree draws nourishment through its roots, and light through its multi-stemmed crown, so we draw *prana* into ourselves mostly as breath through the complex structure of our lungs (which are made up of as many tiny alveoli as there are leaves on a tree), and also through food, and even through our sense organs.

Apana describes the energy that we get rid of, and in so doing give back to our environment, just as a tree gives out different gases, dead leaves and other substances that then become food or compost for other living species. In humans, *apana* is therefore mostly found in the intestines where the metabolic residues are turned into compost. *Apana* is also in our urine and sweat, and in our exhalation; interestingly it is also in much of what we give out as words, and even thoughts.

Both of these energies, *prana* and *apana*, flow up and down the human body in two delicate channels, which curl around the spinal column in spirals, just as the channels that carry the subtle energy currents of trees are described by psychics. The life-enhancing energy of *prana* flows through pingala, the sun channel, which starts at the bottom of and to the right of the spine. The expulsive energy of *apana* flows through *Ida*, the moon channel, which begins to the left and at the bottom of the spine.

According to Yogi Bhajan, these two energies don't meet as long as the person remains fixed in their everyday consciousness. They continue to move up and down, and flow past each other, but never normally come into contact with each other.

Through yogic techniques such as a combination of breathing (*prana*) and pelvic floor exercises (*apana*), the two energies can be stimulated to meet one another. If this happens, an intense inner light in the region of the navel appears. This is the so-called white fire. It is not hot, but is very bright. When this light reaches a certain intensity it flows down two channels, called *reserve-channels*, towards the root chakra at the bottom of the spine. This is how the three and a half coils of Kundalini energy that lie around the root chakra are awakened.

This unified energy then starts to rise up the *Sushumna* central channel. Its clear ascent can be obstructed by what is known in the ancient teachings as *the three knots* or *Granthis*. The first knot, *Brahma Granthi*, is connected with the first and second chakra. It is caused by problems dealing with the material world and the search for sensual satisfaction. The second block, *Vishnu Granthi*, is connected to the third and forth energy centres. For the Kundalini energy to pass through here, the person has to be at peace in dealing with both power and love. The third knot is called *Rudra Granthi*. It is connected to the fifth and sixth charkas, and our ability to communicate, and our readiness to let go of our small and restricted sense of self: the ego.

When these three obstacles are overcome, Kundalini reaches the crown chakra, also known as the lotus of a thousand petals. Notice the tree symbology. This is how the mystical union of root and crown is achieved, and the human being becomes enlightened. Enlightenment generates an expanded state of consciousness, which is physiologically experienced as the release of mood-enhancing hormones. Yogic philosophy symbolically portrays this as a cup brimming with nectar, which overflows in Kundalini awakening. Metaphorically speaking, this ecstasy-bringing nectar drips down to the sixth chakra, giving wings to the intuition, and then down to the heart where a motiveless and unconditional form of love begins to flower. The nectar is also diffused into the aura, the protective magnetic field that envelops the human body, causing it to radiate light.

Trees: A Yogic Perspective

The yogic world-view, like all human attempts to understand the world, does so using human concepts and ideas. From this perspective, trees and humans, and ultimately the entire cosmos, all come from the deific source of all being, known as *Brahma*, 'at one with the all'; and in his perfection he creates the endlessly branching World Tree through *Nada*, the pure stream of sound. The first duality that comes into existence is *Shiva* and *Shakti*, which we would call spirit and nature. *Shiva* represents divine intelligence, enlightened vision, and sometimes a form of wild insanity. Symbolically *Shiva* is portrayed as the eternally dancing deity, who dances so wildly that little drops of light fly from him to become the souls of all life forms. *Shakti*, the nourishing, patient, and at times terrible force of nature, catches these souls and clothes them in bodies made from the five elements of earth, water, fire, air and ether.

The soul particles that *Shakti* has caught are known as *devas*. They travel through a cycle of endless manifestation. Once the source has divided itself to become *Shiva* and *Shakti*, these two energies then come together to form what, from a human perspective, are the 'coarsest' type of things: planets, and all structures made of minerals, such as mountains, deserts, stone, sand; the sun and everything that contains fire, warmth, and light, lightning or magma; the atmosphere and all gaseous aspects of the universe; oceans, and all bodies of water including lakes, rivers, clouds, rain, snow and ice; and finally ether, the invisible world of ideas and formative impulses. Everything is loved and

everything is sacred. *Shiva* and *Shakti* are everywhere, manifest-
ing as different forms.

Having separated from *Brahma*, souls evolve as individuals in
this ultimate play of energies. Yet even at the beginning there is an
impulse and attempt to return to unity.

It is this endeavour by *Shiva* and *Shakti* to melt into each other
and become one that brings into being the second phase of this
cosmic dance. *Shiva* and *Shakti* come closer to one another and
Shiva is no longer pure consciousness, but shows himself as
emotions like longing, fear, sadness, happiness and desire. *Shakti*
is no longer pure form, becoming a changing, striving and repro-
ductive substance. Soul reaches the plant kingdom – the emotional
kingdom.

Along with the famous experiments of connecting plants to lie
detectors,* the phenomenal success of Bach Flower Remedies is
further evidence of the sensitivity and emotional life of plants.
The view of Dr Bach was that every plant, and therefore tree,
strongly embodies one particular emotion. He said, for example,
that the signature energy of the trembling aspen tree is great sensitivity and premonition; while the thick and dark ceiling of leaves
that is the horse chestnut is the embodiment of a protective, yet
also slightly oppressive form of love. The positive effects of Bach
Flower Remedies experienced by countless people prove the
depth of his understanding, and speak volumes for the powerful
interrelationship between plants and emotions.

---

* A good introduction is *The Secret Life of Plants* by Peter Tompkins and
Christopher Bird.

As people, we can also have first-hand experiences of the emotional life of plants. The mere presence of a plant or tree can strengthen or even trigger a depth of feeling, which we may not have discovered otherwise.

Above all, trees can help us to commune with the deepest levels within us, bringing us to a complete unfolding of our consciousness, which has always been the specific concern of Yoga.

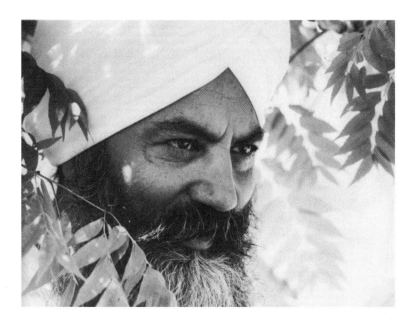

Yogi Bhajan

The young yogi sits high up in the branches of a large Pipal tree. He has been there for three days. When he gets hungry he eats a couple of budding leaves, and in the mornings he licks the dew from the shimmering leaves. At night he goes to a large branch and sleeps there. He even relieves himself somewhere within this broad crown of branches.

It is now the evening of the third day and his master comes strolling back towards him. The yogi quickly gets his best shoes down from a fork in a branch where he has put them so that they don't get dirty, and climbs down. Without letting a word pass his lips about this test of his resolve, he joins the man who has a severe yet noble face, and together they walk back to the village.

The young man was Harbhajan Singh, later known as Yogi Bhajan, master of Kundalini Yoga for about sixty years. He often spoke about the day that, as they were out walking, his Master, Sant Hazara Singh, suddenly told him to climb up a tree and wait there until he came back. This was one of many tasks set him as part of his spiritual education.

Yogi Bhajan was born in Kot Harkarn, in what is now Pakistan, in 1929. By the age of 16 he was already declared a Kundalini master. He often travelled to the Himalayas, and also spent time studying in many different Hatha Yoga ashrams. In 1969 he was invited to Canada by the University of Toronto to teach Yoga. His path then took him to Los Angeles, and from there Kundalini Yoga spread across the whole world.

His three days in the tree stayed with him, and over and again he sent his own students to spend time with trees. It wasn't so much their sacredness in a religious sense, according to the traditional honouring of the Bodhi in Hinduism or the ber tree (also called jujube, Indian plum, or desert apple, *Ziziphus mauritiana*) from Sikh Dharma, but rather an interest in the practical, spiritual teachings from nature:

'The best way to improve your ability to communicate is to walk to a tree and have a chat about what is going on for you. First find a tree standing in a remote place. Now tell the tree about yourself, and then listen to the tree's answer.

Is the giant sequoia not alive? Does it not grow at its own speed? Does it not have its own identity, its own form? Can you speak with the ocean? Can you speak with the wind? Perhaps you think that would be an insane thing to do? No it isn't! We are insane, because we haven't learnt how to speak with the whole world that God created.'
(17. Nov. 1989)

Communication with Trees

At seminars on yoga and communication, which form part of the Kundalini yoga teacher training, we are delighted time and again to find that some of the participants already regularly communicate with trees. Many people spontaneously start talking with trees. This communication can take place at many different levels. Some people even seem able to talk with the Devas (soul beings) of trees. With others, such communication appears to be merely about the projection of an ideal onto the tree. It can also happen that the communication occurs as an intuitive impulse from the person's own subconscious mind, or indeed as a message from their higher-self. Regardless, it is through contact with the tree that such realisations take place, realisations that may not have happened otherwise and then wouldn't be available to the person to increase their self-knowledge.

Added to this there is the art of reading the habit of a tree, which can say so much to those that know how to read it. Is the tree big or small, multi-stemmed or single stemmed? Did it shoot up or grow very slowly? Has it been wounded, and if so how did those wounds heal? Is it infested by parasites, or perhaps full of insects, or visited by birds and other animals? Is it alone or part of a group of other trees? The thing to remember is that each method of understanding has its place and none excludes any other.

You may find the following helpful in your communication with trees:

- Open yourself to your higher consciousness with a few deep breaths, by saying a mantra or affirmation.
- Listen deep within yourself. What would you like to happen through this conversation? What is it that you need?
- Attune yourself to the tree you are with. It is 'awake'? Does it want to talk with you? What does it need?
- Simply enjoy spending some time together in stillness. Then say thanks and goodbye; perhaps leave a present, a beautiful feather or flower, or a spoken mantra.

If you want to ask the tree for advice:

- See if you can describe the situation that you need help with as neutrally as possible, without judging things to be one way or the other.
- Describe your needs, and the feelings you have at this moment.
- Remain in an alert state of stillness; and sensing your togetherness with the tree, open yourself to everything that is, giving thanks for the way you feel, however you feel. Emotions want to be felt, to enable you to recognise what it really is that you need. As soon as you recognise this you will feel a lightness, and the path towards a solution will come to you.
- To end with, thank the tree; again, take a few deep breaths, or say a mantra, or blessing. Leave a loving energy behind you as you say your goodbyes.

Part II

Asana

'Look at a tree, a flower, a plant.
Let your awareness rest upon it.
How still they are, how deeply rooted in Being.
Allow nature to teach you stillness.
When you look at a tree and perceive its still-
ness, you become still yourself.
You connect with it at a very deep level.
You feel a oneness with whatever you perceive
in and through stillness.
Feeling the oneness of yourself with all things
is true love.'

Eckhart Tolle

From the book *Stillness Speaks,* Copyright 2003 by
Eckhart Tolle. Reprinted with permission of New World
Library, Novato, CA. www.newworldlibrary.com

To attune to a tree:
Stand upright in front of it,
feet about 50 cm apart.
Stretch your arms up,
spread your fingers,
and face your open palms forwards.

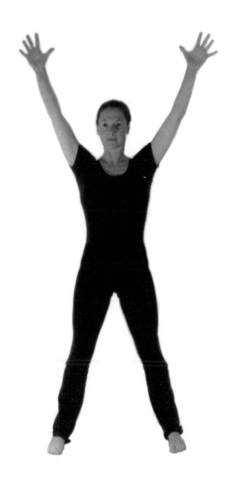

Tree Yoga

'The first time we went to practice yoga under a tree I was really tired, not a good place from which to start practicing yoga. It was springtime, and somewhat reticently we stood before a young, vibrantly green, pine tree. This pine was a little removed from the rest of the trees and its cone-bearing branches were dancing lightly in the breeze. At first we didn't notice anything particularly unusual. We performed our exercises, and then, after a little pause, sat ourselves down to meditate. Suddenly, like a breaking wave, a feeling of happiness and power came over our little group, in a way that I have seldom experienced. My exhaustion was swept away, and we all agreed that the tree had infected us all with its vibrancy, awakening our joie de vivre.'

Satya Singh

As will become clear during the rest of this book, and as already introduced, every species of tree embodies particular qualities and energies, and has its own voice. In general terms, for example, the pine is a spirited warrior, full of vigour. The beech exudes stability and discipline, while the elm supports our ability to communicate. So it makes sense to practice exercises that give us courage under a pine, and exercises to help us to be grounded and help our clarity under a beech. The tree and the qualities that it radiates will support us in realising such goals.

Our initial idea with tree yoga is to first decide which exercises you want to do, and then go outside to find a tree whose energies will support the intention behind the exercises you have chosen. If possible, practice them under, or at least nearby, the tree that you find. To help you identify the trees in this book, we have included photos and close-up illustrations.

Another way of working with tree yoga is just to go outside and find one of the twelve species included in this book, one that grabs your attention, and then carry out the exercises suggested for that particular species.

Of course, if neither of the above is possible, you can always do the exercises at home and visualise the type of tree that you want to work with. Imagination can sometimes create the same effects as reality.

A fourth way to work with tree yoga is to go outside and find a tree that you feel connected to, regardless of whether it is one of the twelve trees included in the book. Spend some time and try to get a sense of your chosen tree's energies, and then perform the exercises from the book that go with those energies.

The sequences that have been put together in this book all come from Yogi Bhajan's Kundalini Yoga. None of them are Kriyas in the sense that they have to be done in strict order. Rather, any exercise that we give here can happily be done on its own. If you feel inspired to know more about Kundalini Yoga, you will find a complete description and introduction in: *Kundalini Yoga: A Simple Guide to the Yoga of Awareness: The Flow of Eternal Power: A Simple Guide to the Yoga of Awareness as Taught by Yogi Bhajan, Ph. D.* by Shakti Parwha Kaur Khalsa, Penguin Group 1998. Or chose one of the titles given at the end of this book.

Preparation

- It is important to do tree yoga, (or any type of yoga) on an empty stomach. So, bearing that in mind, don't eat for two to three hours beforehand.

- Before, during, and after doing yoga, drink plenty of water. You could bring a bottle of still mineral water with you, and every now and again take a few sips. Water aids the physical, emotional and spiritual cleansing that is initiated by the exercises.

- Be careful not to get cold during the exercises. This is particularly important when it comes to the relaxation and meditation. Take your meditation shawl or a blanket, and during the relaxation you can use it to cover yourself. Then you can put it around your shoulders during the meditation.

- If you want to sit to meditate (it is possible to meditate standing up but sitting usually works much better), the best thing is to use a sheepskin to sit on or something else made from a natural material. You could use a folded woollen blanket or raffia mat. Synthetic fibres or materials have a strongly disturbing effect on our bodies and the voltage of the air around us. They are best avoided because they inhibit the flow of naturally-generated energetic fields, and in the forest act to insulate you from the living soil.

- Wear loose fitting clothing, best made from organic cotton or linen.

- If you are having treatment for back problems or other health issues, please get in touch with your healthcare professional and check that the exercises in this book are suitable for you. Even if you are given the go-ahead, do take care not to overstep your comfort zone. If you have had slipped discs in the past, take particular care with exercises where you are being asked to bend forwards. A good rule of thumb in this case is to contract your pelvic floor whenever you are bending forwards or backwards. (See p. 48 on Bandhas.)

- Menstruating women should take particular care to listen to their bodies. As a general rule it is better not to do any strong exercises that put pressure on the abdominal muscles.

- Yoga exercises are traditionally done barefoot, to allow the feet to breathe. But if it's too cold or dirty, just leave your shoes on.

The Basics

Attunement

Before beginning, attune yourself by singing ONG NAMO GURUDEV NAMO three times. This means: 'I greet the cosmic energy and the exalted path that leads from the darkness into the light.' Hold each tone for a while, and although you have your mouth open, allow most of your breath, and most of the sound too, to flow out of your nostrils. This will make the roof of your mouth vibrate, positively influencing the hypothalamus and pituitary glands in your brain. (See *Mantras* below.)

Breath

Long, deep breathing. The breath begins by extending the abdominal wall (1), then the ribs widen (2). Lastly the upper chest, collarbones and breastbone get pulled forwards and outwards (3). On the first step of the exhale the upper chest relaxes (3), then the ribs sink (2), and finally the abdominal wall contracts (1). Long, deep breaths are both relaxing and centring.

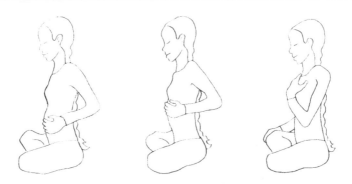

The Breath of Fire is done purely using the abdomen. As you breathe in, quickly extend your belly forwards, and then as you breathe out bring it in again. The illustration shows you how the right hand stays still and the abdominal wall moves the left hand. The ideal Breath of Fire is fast, up to two per second; but start off slowly, you'll get there in your own time.

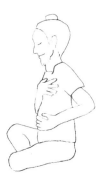

40 days, 90 days, 1000 days
Just practicing yoga as and when you can, you'll really notice the difference. But if you really want to change something about the way life is for you, then follow a series of exercises or do a meditation systematically, every day. The traditional length of time to do this is 40, 90, or 1000 days. In this way, the energies and transformative power that is awoken by the exercises will become ever more deeply anchored in your being.

Mantras
One of the important goals of practicing yoga is to bring to stillness the part of us that is often compared to a ridiculous monkey, because it is so hard to harness its energy. To do this, points of focus both inside and outside the body are used. *Mantras* (words and sounds to accompany meditation) are just that. The main *mantra* in Kundalini yoga is *Sat Nam*. This *mantra* accompanies every breath, even if no *mantra* is mentioned as being part of the exercise. Think *Sat or Saaaaaaat* while breathing in, and *Nam* or *Naaaaaaam*, while breathing out. *Sat* means truth, and *Nam* identity. *Sat Nam* means true identity or *who you really are*. You can hear the *mantra* being sung if you go to: *www.satyasingh.com*

Intensity and length of exercises
Generally do each exercise for 1–3 minutes, unless it says otherwise. Each one of us should determine the intensity with which
we approach a particular exercise. Do it gently enough so as not to
harm yourself, but strongly enough to grow beyond your present
comfort zone.

Mudras
Mudras are special hand or finger positions that are connected
with the reflex areas and meridians found in the hands, and have
a powerful yet subtle effect. The most often used *Mudra* is *Gyan
Mudra*, where the ends of the thumb and forefinger are held
together, while the other fingers are gently stretched outwards.

The thumb is the "I", the ego, and the forefinger is the Jupiter
finger, finger of growth and wisdom.

Points of Focus
Spiritual presence is elevated when two or more points of focus
are used. This might be saying or singing the Mantra, *Sat Nam*,
while focusing on the sense of gravity, or using your eyes to
concentrate on a point on a tree, while at the same time focusing
on your breath.

Bhandas
The *Bhandas* are known as the body's locks. They are made from
muscle but are not used to help the body to move, rather playing
a supportive role as well as having an opening and closing function. They are used in Yoga because they help to bring energy up
the body. There are four of them and they are called:

Mulbhand, the root lock, is part of the pelvic floor musculature. To engage this lock you pull in the muscles around the anus, sexual organs and lower abdomen. For women the centre of this contraction is the mouth of the uterus. For men it is the perineum, between the anus and penis. In principle, *Mulbhand* can be engaged after every exercise, and especially at the end of each meditation. To do this, take a deep breath and hold it for 10 seconds while pulling up the *Mulbhand*, letting go as you breathe out. Do this once or twice, as you like. *Mulbhand* directs the energy in the abdominal cavity upwards, as well as having lots of other benefits, including on the blood pressure and lymph system. Any time that you are intensively bending your torso, it's a good idea to lightly engage the *Mulbhand* to support your spine.

Uddhyana Bhand, the diaphragm lock, is activated when you contract your abdomen and draw it upwards. Doing this transports the energy in the chest upwards.

Jalandhara Bhand, the neck lock, elevates the neck vertebra. Engage this lock by pulling in your chin, while at the same time pulling up the top of your head. Don't bend your head forwards at the same time. You will notice that your chest lifts slightly as you do this. This *Bhand* allows energy to flow into your head unhindered.

Maha Bhand, the great lock, is engaged by using all three of the others together, while at the same time bringing your tongue backwards and pressing it onto your soft pallet, and also closing your eyes and rolling your eyeballs upwards. This *Bhanda* is often used at the end of an exercise or meditation. To do it, first breathe out, and stop yourself from breathing in again for 10 seconds, while engaging the *Maha Bhand*. This means pulling up your pelvic floor, pulling in your abdomen and drawing it up, pulling in your chin, holding your tongue back and pressing it against the roof of your mouth and rolling your eyes to the ceiling.

Standing Postures

> 'You can learn from a tree to stand in ecstasy.'
>
> Yogi Bhajan

Tree yoga is only made up of standing exercises. The different postures are:

- Hip-width: feet about 30 cm apart, parallel to one another.

- Shoulder-width: feet about 50 cm apart, again parallel to one another.

- Gentle stretch posture: feet about 70 cm apart, and turned slightly outwards.

- Strong stretch posture: feet about 90 cm apart and again turned slightly outwards.

- The Archer: one foot pointing forwards, the other about 75 cm back, turned outwards at a 45-degree angle.

Relaxation

With tree yoga you are quite free to choose your own form of relaxation. Choose for yourself whether and when you need to relax, and whether you do this standing, sitting, or lying down. A good rule of thumb is that if you are doing a series of, say, nine exercises, that you take a rest for one or two minutes after the third and sixth ones. Any longer and the energy wave that you have been building will drop off again. At the end of a series, relax for between ten and fifteen minutes. While relaxing, it's great just to let go of everything. Or, you can listen to the sounds around you, experience the pull of gravity, and acknowledge your breath.

Suitability
If health problems stop you from doing an exercise, like the crouching or crow postures, see if you can change the exercise in a way that makes it possible for you. For example, if doing the crow, turn it into more of a standing pose.

Meditation
The meditation that comes after each tree yoga exercise will deepen its effect. You can decide whether to meditate standing or sitting. As we have said before, sitting is preferable. Sitting is a more stable posture to meditate in, enabling you to go deeper and 'forget' about your body for a while. Of course it is really beautiful to sit with your back to the trunk of the tree, like the Buddha under the pipal or bodhi tree.

BIRCH
(Betula)

The birch tree is loved by all. Its light and graceful presence is uplifting and gives solace in the sometimes dark woodland of the northern hemisphere. The same goes for the homoeopathic remedy, Betula, which brings light where there is darkness.

Birches are pioneers, taking root on fallow land, and preparing the ground for other trees to create a forest. The laid-back stand of birches soon becomes populated and then supplanted by other trees. Birches don't stand their ground, neither geographically nor as individual trees. They very rarely live to be 100 years old and always appear young, never growing into a stiff old age. See the supple birch dancing in the wind and witness its unsurpassable lightness and grace.

In Russia and northern Europe, the traditional power of the birch is one of new beginnings, as told in legends. And this is just what the eternally youthful birch helps us to do, to start again. Look to the seed of its being and you will find the archetype of the great mother, that protects and nourishes everything that is young. With the unconditional love of a mother, the birch blesses all types of love, from the immature love of a teenager to romantic love, and also natural, unashamedly erotic love. Many traditional spring and fertility rites honour the birch (as well as the hawthorn).

At the same time, especially in shamanistic traditions, the birch is the gatekeeper of the spiritual world. After all, stepping into the unseen dimensions, be it through trance, astral-travelling, meditation and even death, is always a new beginning. Wherever it is we are travelling to, regardless of the new horizon we are meeting, the spirit of the birch is here to guide us.

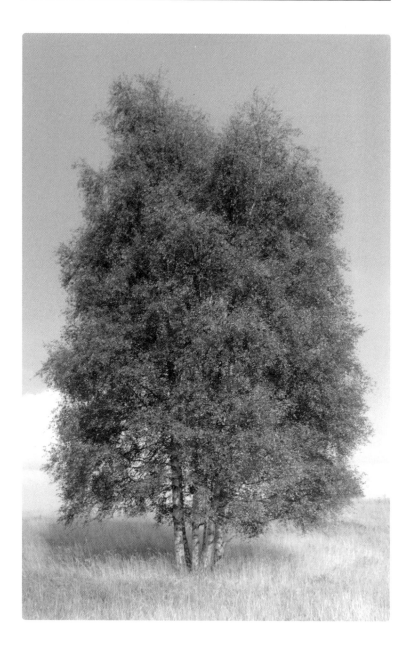

> The key words that attune us to the spiritual home of the birch tree are *new beginnings, protection, innocence* and *the joy of living.*

Exercise Sequence for the Joy of Living

We recommend that you do these exercises under or close to a birch tree. If that's just not possible, as we said in the introduction, visualise a birch tree. The energy of this tree strengthens the effect of these exercises.

The Joy of Living, Part 1

Relaxation through movement:

a) Slowly dance under or around the birch to some nice, soft music. 1–3 minutes.

You could hum, sing, or bring an instrument with you.

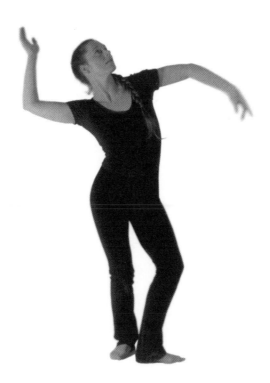

b) Use your hands to gently say hello to your whole body.

c) With your feet shoulder-width apart, bend your upper body backwards, with your arms hanging loosely by your sides. Engage *Mulbhand*. Breathe long and deep. 1 minute.

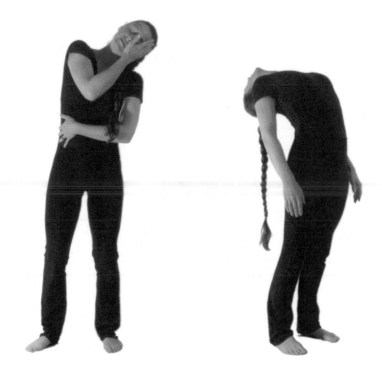

d) With your feet still shoulder-width apart, let your upper body hang down to the front. Again breathe long and deep. 1–3 minutes.

To relax the spine.

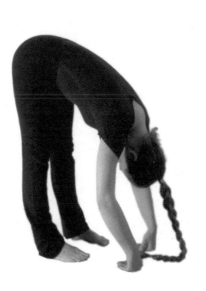

The Joy of Living, Part 2

a) With your feet hip-width apart, hold your arms in front of you at shoulder height. With a wave-like motion, start to move your hands, arms, shoulders, torso, hips and knees.

Now stand on your toes and swing your arms backwards making a circle, and then forwards again. 1–3 minutes.

To loosen and energise.

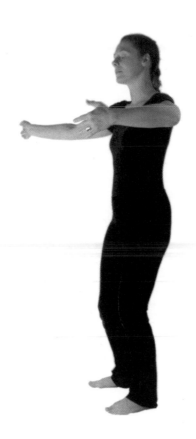

b) Crow posture.

With your feet still hip-width apart, crouch down, keeping the soles of your feet flat on the floor. Stretch your arms straight out in front of you; knit your fingers together and point your fore-fingers. Keep your upper body vertical and breathe long and slow. 1–3 minutes.

The crow posture works on the large intestines, which are psycho-somatically connected to our ability to let go. The forefinger holds the energy of Jupiter, which is associated with being positive.

If you need to, you can put a piece of wood under your heels so that you make contact with the whole of your foot.

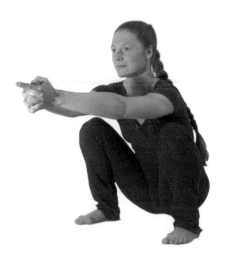

c) While standing, bend down and hold your ankles; now start to walk around while keeping your legs straight. 1 minute.

This stretches the back of your legs, while giving you an unusual perspective of the world.

A slight variation would be to place your hands around your knees or calves.

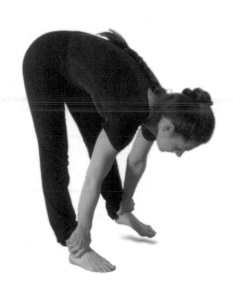

The Joy of Living, Part 3

a) With your feet hip-width apart and your arms by your sides, turn your palms to face the front and breathe in. Make a fist with your left hand; bend your left elbow; and as you breathe out move your fist to your right shoulder, while you turn your whole body to the left. As you breathe in again, bring your fist down again; open your hand, and turn your body back to the centre again. Repeat this movement as you breathe out, with your right fist, turning to the right as you bring your arm to your shoulder. Now that you can do this, bring up your right knee as you turn to the left, and your left knee as you turn to the right. Change sides in swift succession. 3 minutes.

This exercise wakes you up and makes you feel bright and breezy.

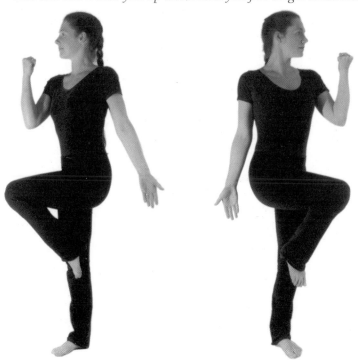

b) Laugh!

Quiet or loud, as you like, using your diaphragm and coming from your belly. 5 minutes.

Laughing heals the heart.

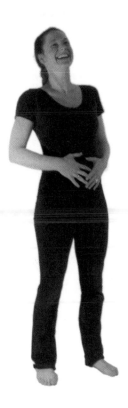

c) Have your feet about 50 cm apart. Now stretch up your arms about 60 degrees apart, with your palms facing the front and your fingers spread out. Long, slow breath. 2 minutes.

Strengthens the heart.

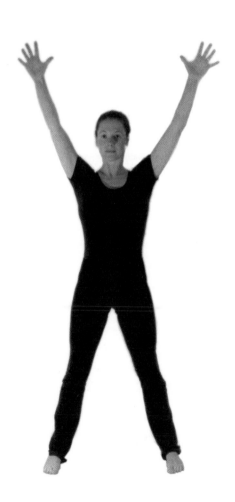

Relaxation
(standing, sitting, or lying down) 1–11 minutes

Listen to the rustling of the leaves, and the all-enveloping stillness.

Meditation for clarity of purpose

(YB 4 Nov. 1975)

Sit easily with your legs crossed. Hold your hands in front of your throat, palms facing you, supporting the one hand with the other; women, right hand above the left; men, left hand above the right. In this way the top edge of the lower hand is pressing into the bottom edge of the upper hand. Using a rhythmical movement, press the thumb of your lower hand into the roots of each finger, starting with the little finger and working your way up. When

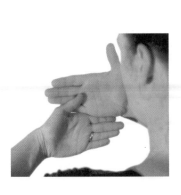
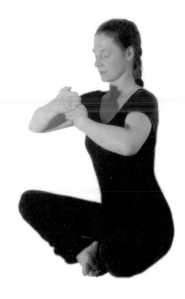

you get to your forefinger, start at the little finger again. Each time you press your thumb, say an affirmation.

An affirmation is a short, positive sentence affirming a reality that you would like to create for yourself. Below we have given you a few examples that fit with the key words belonging to the birch: new beginnings, protection, innocence, and the joy of living.

'I give thanks for the past and am free to create my future.'

'The universe completely protects and supports me.'

'I am happy to be myself.'

Start with 11 minutes a day, and gradually increase to 31 minutes.

Affirmations influence your spirit and subconscious. They work best if they are done daily for a few minutes at a time. Doing them will make it easier for the reality you are affirming to manifest itself.

ELM
(Ulmus)

Elms grow all over the world. Along with oaks, beech, limes and black poplars, they belong to the great deciduous trees.

The elm has long played a many-sided role in the daily lives of human beings. As far back as the Stone Age, its leaves were being used as animal fodder. And its biological rhythm has long been used by farmers as a reliable indicator for correct planting times.

Spiritually the elm's power is communication, and for us that means communication with other kingdoms of nature; so through its presence, communication with animals, plants, nature spirits and our ancestors can take place. Both in ancient Britain and classical Greece, the elm was used in death rituals. An old English name is *elven wood*, pointing to its connection with nature spirits.

After Orpheus lost his beloved Eurydice, he courageously travelled into the underworld and wrestled her from Hades (god of the underworld), only to lose her again at the last moment. As he sat defeated under the elm tree, he took up his harp and played such an enchanting song of unutterable grief and despair that all the woodland animals gathered around him, and even the wind held its breath.

Between 1960 and 1990 most fully grown elms were killed off by Dutch Elm Disease. The cause of this is found in a fungus, spread from tree to tree by a beetle that lays its eggs under the bark of the elm tree. Millions of young elm trees survived, but as soon as a tree reaches a certain size and thickness of bark, the fungus attacks it again. Because of this illness it is as though the elm is frozen in time, destined never to fully become itself.

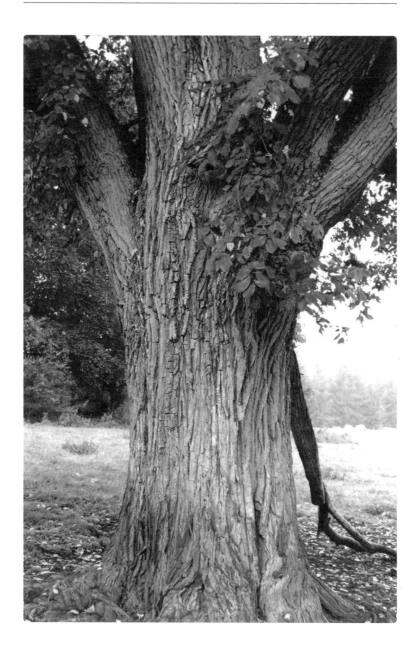

If we come from the perspective that all beings are inter-connected and that the physical world is a mirror of the spiritual world, then the desperate state of the elm is to a certain extent a reflection of our collective form of communication. Communication in modern society denies the possibility of communicating with the other kingdoms of nature and is limited to the total exploitation of plants, animals and natural resources. The material and rational worldview dominates and also marginalises elderly people and their wisdom, creating a cultural hegemony in which, for example, discussion of death and afterlife are completely taboo. Elms die in a world in which free and open communication is rapidly dying, communication that is replaced with anonymous information delivery and questionnaires.

Without a living exchange, information stays superficial and doesn't nourish the soul. The possibility of experiencing our unity within creation, and our interconnectedness with all beings, is actually available to us in each moment, and the elm can help us.

> The key words to attune ourselves to the spirit of the elm tree are *communication, love, letting go,* and *freedom.*

Exercise Sequence to Learn How to Let Go

We recommend doing these exercises underneath or in view of an elm tree. If that isn't possible, visualise an elm tree in front of you. The energy of the tree strengthens the effect of the exercises.

Letting Go, Part 1 (shankasana series)

a) Have your feet hip-width apart. Place your right hand on your right hip, fingers facing backwards, thumb facing forwards. Bring your left hand behind your back and take hold of your right wrist. Turn your whole body to the left as you breathe in, and then to the right as you breathe out. Your feet stay flat on the ground. With your eyes shut, direct your eyes as if you were looking between the centre of your eyebrows. 1 minute.

Then change hands and turn to the right. 1 minute.

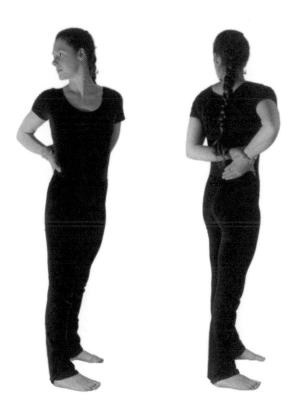

b) With your feet hip-width apart, put both hands on your hips, thumbs pointing forwards. Pull back your elbows so that your shoulder blades are pulled together. As you breathe in, turn your whole body to the left, and then to the right as you breathe out. Keep your feet flat on the floor, and your eyes closed. With closed eyelids, turn your eyes as if you were looking at the central point between your eyebrows. 1 minute.

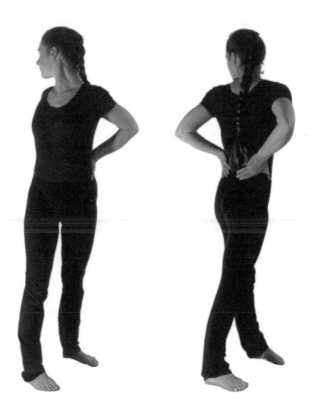

c) Again, feet hip-width apart. Put your arms behind your back, palms facing your lower back, now interlock your fingers. Tighten your pelvic floor muscles and move your upper body in large circles, breathing in as you circle backwards, and out as you circle forwards. With closed eyelids, turn your eyes as if you were looking at the central point between your eyebrows. 1 minute.

Shankasana means posture of the conch-shell.

It cleanses the liver and kidneys, and keeps the spine supple.

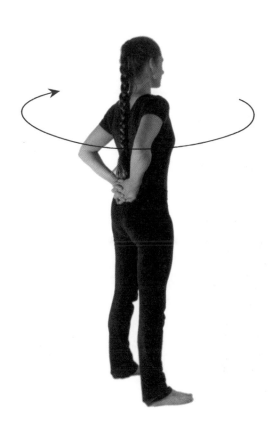

Letting Go, Part 2

a) Place your feet about 90 cm apart; breathe in deeply, and stretch your arms over your head, bringing your palms together. Tighten your pelvic floor; breathe out and bend forwards putting both hands on your left foot or shinbone. Stay in this position while you practice the Breath of Fire (see p. 47). Keep your legs stretched, your back straight and your eyes closed. 1–3 minutes.

Now tighten your pelvic floor again and breathe in as you bring yourself back up. Stretch up once; and then as you breathe out and hold your pelvic floor, bend down to your right foot. Again stay in that position while doing the Breath of Fire. 1–3 minutes.

This stretches the so-called sexual nerve, responsible for your vitality, freedom and flexibility.

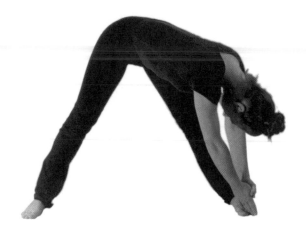

b) Bring your feet to hip-width apart, and touch the ends of your thumbs and little fingers together. Now, as you breathe in, stretch your arms forwards and upwards with palms downwards, making a big circular movement until your hands are high above your head. Breathe out as you bring your arms backwards and down again. Keep your arms straight, and with closed eyelids turn your eyes as if you were looking at the central point between your eyebrows. 4–5 minutes.

The little finger is related to the planet Mercury, meaning that this Mudra, or hand position, de- velops *our communication skills.*

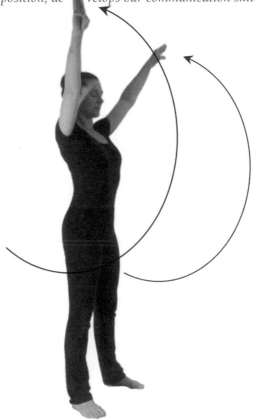

Letting Go, Part 3

a) With your feet hip-width apart, let your arms loosely hang by your sides. Lift your chin and stretch your neck without letting your head fall backwards. Take long deep breaths. 1–3 minutes.

This strengthens your voice, and throat chakra.

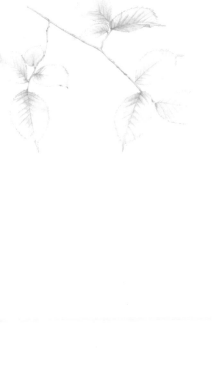

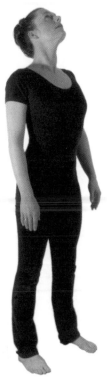

b) Stand upright with your feet hip-width apart.

1) Purse your lips and suck in your breath.

2) Holding your breath, push out your cheeks.

3) Put your thumbs in your ears, forefingers over your eyes, pushing your nostrils shut with your middle and ring fingers.

4) Bend your head forwards, stretching your neck.

5) Hold your breath for as long as you can.

6) Bring your head back up and breathe out through pursed lips.

Repeat the above sequence for 1–3 minutes.

This exercise sharpens the perception by strengthening the eyes and ears.

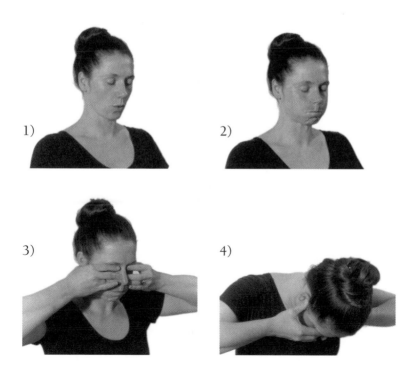

1)

2)

3)

4)

c) Stand with your feet hip-width apart. Tighten your pelvic floor, bending your torso forwards while holding your back straight; keep going until your back is parallel to the floor. Let your arms and hands dangle while holding up your head and keeping your eyes closed. Stay in this posture and start singing a mantra or song. You could sing Oooooong, which is the primal sound, or we could call it creational energy of the cosmos. 1–3 minutes.

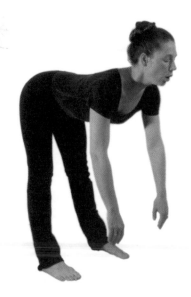

Relaxation
(while standing, sitting or lying down) 1–11 minutes
Listen to the sound of the leaves rustling and the stillness in-between.

Meditation to develop the art of speaking consciously

(Yogi Bhajan, Spain 1986)

Sit easily, legs crossed, and put your hands on your knees in the Gyan Mudra (see p. 48). Keep your elbows straight, and in tune with the rhythm of your heart start to sing the mantra: MAA MAA MAA MAA MAA MAA... Your lips will start to tingle after a while. (Listen to this mantra at www.satyasingh.com/treeyoga)

You have three points of focus:

your lips,

the sound and,

your third eye (the point between your eyebrows).

Sing the mantra for 3,11 or 31 minutes.

'MAA' is the first word that every baby thinks and speaks. Because of this it is instilled deeply within our subconscious, and using it as a mantra has a very healing and integrating effect.

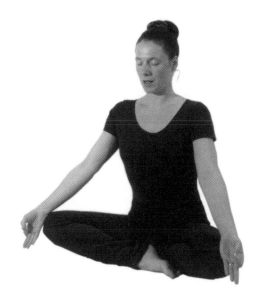

WHITE WILLOW

(Salix alba)

Throughout all times and cultures the willow has been connected to the feminine, the moon, and the element of water in all its
forms. Many of the goddesses of the ancient world resided in
sacred willows or willow groves. For the Sumerians, for example,
this goddess was Belili, who ruled the moon, love, sexuality, and
the underworld, and was worshipped where there were willows,
springs and wells. In classical Greece the willow was dedicated to
Persephone, goddess of the underworld, and Kirke, who weaves
and sings at the navel of the world.

The same association of the feminine and the willow is seen
in Celtic tradition. In ancient Scotland, the willow represented
strength and harmony. The later kings of the Scottish Isles, and
the chieftains of the more powerful clans, would hold a branch
of willow while administering justice – a custom that is a vivid
reminder of the matriarchal structures that influenced the Celts.

Even in Christian times, this tree remained anchored in folklore. There are countless numbers of invocations and little rituals
designed to invoke the magic of this tree to dispel pain or mis-
fortune, and especially infertility. Much is based on superstition,
but not all is a game of smoke and mirrors, not by any stretch of
the imagination. Willow has many practical medicinal qualities.
Salicin, which is found in the bark, is a natural painkiller that has
been synthesised since 1898, and is still used today as an ingre-
dient in painkillers.

The rituals performed by witch covens became centred on the
willow tree, and as a result the willow became a focus for the
hatred of Christian missionaries. Later on, in the mythological

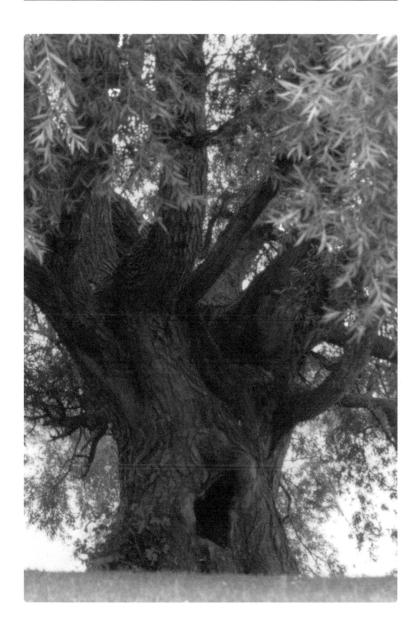

writings of the 19th and 20th centuries, the willow is often associated with grief and sadness. The only basis for this interpretation is the biblical Psalm 137 where it is said that the exiled Hebrews, when they had given up all hope, hung their harps from the branches of 'willow' trees by the 'waters of Babylon'. Thinking of this, Christian botanists named a species of willow they had imported from Asia 'weeping willow' (*Salix babylonica*) because of its hanging branches. Hence the connection between the willow and grief, which is an historical misinterpretation. Actually it was the reverse, as we see when Yahweh, the God of the Old Testament orders that the tabernacle be joyously decorated with branches of willow. It's also worth noting that the 'weeping willow' of the Babylonian exiles was actually a type of poplar!

It is interesting that so much superstition and misinterpretation surrounds the willow. One reason for this may be that one of the associations of the moon, with which the willow is intimately connected, is that of illusion. Think if you will of the the Moon tarot card, the card of illusion. The flowing willow has soft, blurred edges, and an equally blurred identity, with flowing boundaries between it and its surroundings. This is very noticeable if you compare its form to the sharp and edgy contours (and history) of the oak, for example.

Putting human error to one side, we see that the willow is a tree of remarkable vitality and fertility. Single cut twigs of willow put out new roots and grow into trees themselves if just heeled into wet ground. Damaged branches can also recover to become dense thickets. The incredible regenerative abilities of the willow would no doubt make it immortal were it not for the fact that its quick growing and soft wood is so susceptible to fungal growth.

Willow teaches us to focus our energy in the here and now, and dive into the flow of life, without holding back, so that old wounds can heal and new growth can take place.

> The key words that attune us to the spiritual realm of the willow are *flowing*, *openness*, and *being at home in oneself*.

Exercise Sequence to Increase Flexibility

We recommend doing these exercises under or in view of a willow tree. If that isn't possible, visualise a willow instead. The energy of the tree strengthens the effect of the exercises.

Flexibility, Part 1

a) Stand up straight and stretch your left arm horizontally to the left. As you breathe in, lift your right leg to the side, as high as you can. Let it down slowly again as you breathe out. Your arm should stay horizontal. 2 minutes. Don't change sides, this exercise is designed just to be done like this.

Stimulates the brain and stretches the right sciatic nerve.

b) Place your feet hip-width apart; as you breathe out, take your arm in a curve over your head while bending down to the right. At the same time see how far towards the ground your right arm can slide down your leg. Breathe in, straighten, breathe out and repeat the exercise on the other side. Watch out that you don't bend forwards or backwards. 25 times on each side.

Stretches the main back muscles and intercostal muscles (important for breathing).

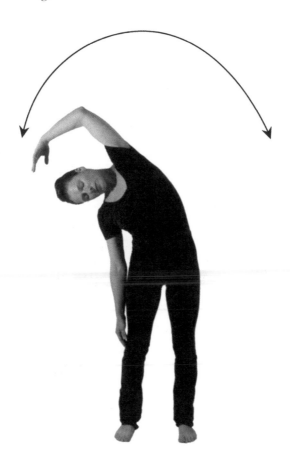

c) Place your feet hip-width apart, stand tall and pull up your pelvic floor muscles. Clasp your hands behind your back. As you breathe in, lift your chest, bend your neck and bend backwards, stretching your arms downwards and away from your body. Then as you breathe out keeping your pelvic floor contracted, bend forwards, bringing your head down towards your knees and stretch your arms away from your body.

Increases the flexibility of the thoracic vertebrae.

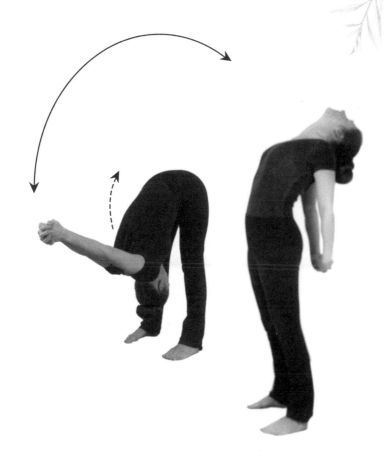

Flexibility, Part 2

a) Bend down and place both hands just above your right knee.
With a straight back, stretch your left leg to the back so that your
leg and upper body are horizontal to the ground. Breathe long
and deep. Keep your eyes focused on one point on the ground to
help keep your balance. 1 minute 30 seconds, then change sides.

*This exercise enhances balance and reduces the chance of degener-
ative disease developing.*

You can support yourself on the tree or a wall.

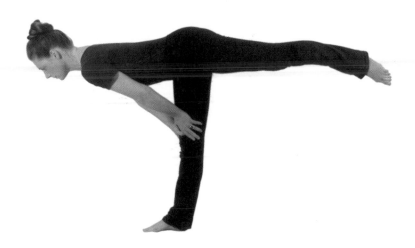

b) Assume the crouching pose. (Feet hip-width or slightly more apart, heels flat on the floor, back of the head elevated.) Place your hands around your ankles. As you breathe in, stretch your legs bringing your head towards your knees. As you breathe out, come back to crouching again. 2 minutes.

You may want to place your hands just above your knees and just bring your bottom down as far as you can.

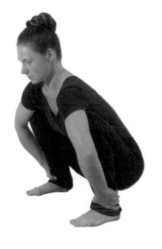

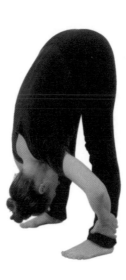

c) Place your feet as wide apart as you can (about 90 cm or so); support your hands on your hips with your fingers pointing backwards and your thumbs forwards. Tense your pelvic floor muscles, lift your chest, and bend backwards as far as possible as you breathe in. As you breathe out, bend forwards and see if you can touch the ground with your head. 1–3 minutes.

Bending forwards is about being able to humble yourself.

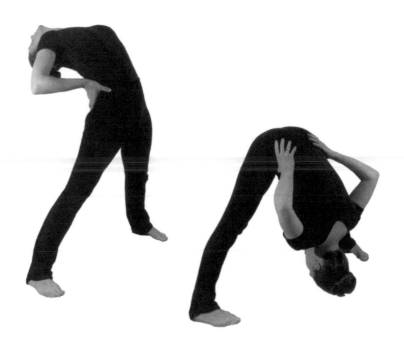

Flexibility, Part 3

a) Place your feet hip-width apart and stretch your arms over your head, palms facing forwards. Keep your pelvic floor elevated, lift your chest, and bend your upper body as far back as you can. Close your eyes. Firebreathe (p. 47). 1–3 minutes.

The ability to bend backwards is to do with trust, being able to open yourself and give service. This pose strongly exercises the forth thoracic vertebra and is good therapy for asthma sufferers.

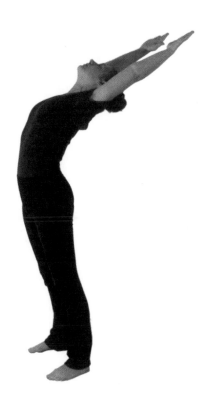

b) Place your feet about 50 cm apart. Stretch up your arms up so that they are about 60 degrees apart; your palms are open and face the front. Spread your fingers wide and shut your eyes. Long, deep breaths. 2 minutes.

Attune yourself even deeper to the tree.

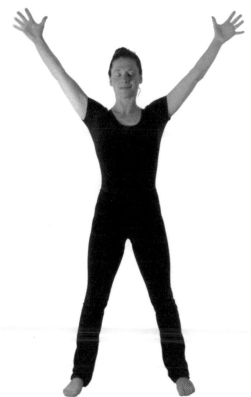

Relaxation
(standing, sitting, or lying) 1–11 minutes
Listen to the murmuring of the leaves and branches, and the stillness that envelops everything.

Meditation for health and wellbeing

(YB 3 March 1978)

Sit with your legs crossed and hold your hands at the level of your diaphragm in the *Shambavi Mudra*. Your right hand palm up, lying in your left hand, with your left thumb lying in the palm of your right hand, and right thumb resting on left thumb. Let your breath flow in and out freely. Your eyes are open about 1/10, your gaze directed to the end of your nose.

Keeping your eyes about 1/10 open helps you to stay present and not drift away in this meditation.

'As soon as you start holding this pose you'll start to feel very comfortable in yourself.

As you become the seed at the centre of life, nature will start to serve you. This is the easiest way to live in harmony.

See if you can break through the barriers of time and space. The same energy that prevents us can also help us to break through.' (Yogi Bhajan)

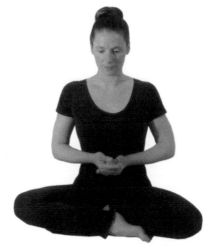

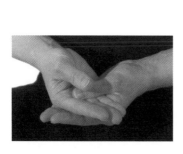

CEDAR OF LEBANON
(Cedrus libani)

The oldest descriptions that we have of the cedar of Lebanon being a sacred tree come from the Near East, especially from what used to be Mesopotamia. Over 5,000 years ago the Sumerians saw the World Tree as rooted within the centre of the earth, its crown said to carry the primordial heavens on its branches. The World Tree nourishes all of life; its innermost core is a temple too sacred for mortal life to step within. For the Babylonians, heirs of Sumerian culture, this was the dwelling place of the cosmic mother, Ishtar, and her divine son, Tammuz.

The cedar of Lebanon was regarded as the representative of the World Tree on the earthly plane. In its heart lived Ea, deity of wisdom and source of the forces behind civilisation: laws and moral codes, healing, trade, literature, art and science. This is particularly meaningful as Mesopotamia is widely regarded as the cradle of civilization.

Many hundreds of years later, in the same area, the Chaldaeans still upheld the sacred cedar rituals 'to invigorate and strengthen the life force of the body'. They invoked the spirit of the cedar as the 'oracle of heaven and earth.'

In the 10ᵗʰ century BC, King Solomon built the legendary Temple of Jerusalem. He took what appeared to many to be un-reasonable steps to ensure that the main construction was built using wood from the cedar of Lebanon, a material both coveted and very famous in the Old World. (The Lebanon is a chain of mountains in the Phoenician hinterland, bordering Israel and Judaea to the north.) Solomon traded whole border territories of his kingdom with the Phoenicians to gain the precious wood he wanted for his temple. Once he had built his temple, he decorated it with numerous images of the Tree of Life.

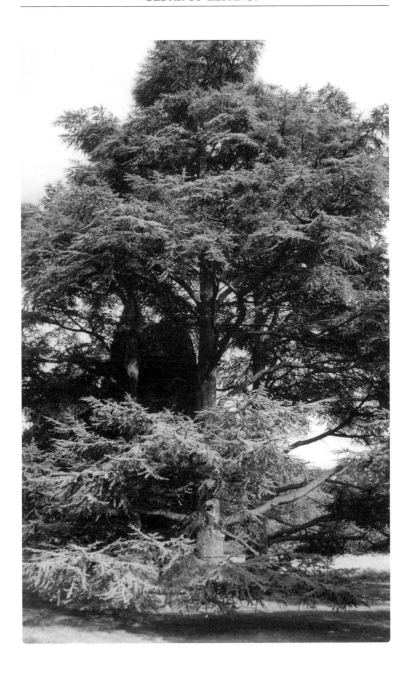

Still today, the cedar takes a very special place in the spiritual traditions of the indigenous peoples of North America. The cedar is the wood of choice for totem poles on the northern coasts of America and Canada.*

It is fascinating to discover that the oldest religious text discovered to date is also an ecological warning. The Sumerian Gilgamesh epic tells the story of Gilgamesh's small-minded and desperate search for deification and immortality. In the process of trying to fulfil his ambitions, he destroys a sacred grove in a virgin cedar forest. His attack on nature leads not only to his own ruin, but also to the death of his only friend. Surely as clear a warning as we can have not to exploit woodland for our own selfish ends.

The teaching of the cedar has been the same since the beginning of civilisation: don't try to separate the needs of the ego (the small self that cares for our own survival) from the needs of the earth, who is our greater self and cares for the survival of all. What we do to the one, we do to the other.

> The key words to attune yourself to the spirit of the cedar are *inner majesty, grace* and *indestructibility.*

Exercise Sequence to Encourage Grace

We recommend that you carry out these exercises either under or in view of a cedar tree. If that's not possible, you can visualise a cedar. The energy of the tree strengthens the effect of the exercises.

---

* Botanically speaking, most American cedars are actually cypresses or false cypresses. For more information on this see Fred's book *The Living Wisdom of Trees*, chapter Cedar.

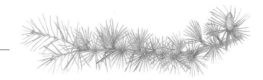

Grace, Part 1

a) Place your feet shoulder-width apart. Bend your knees a little and put your hands on your thighs. Breathe in deep and slow; now hold your breath for a moment and then push out your belly. Then breathe out slowly, again hold your breath for a moment and then pull your belly in and upwards with your diaphragm until there is a large space where your belly used to be. This movement works the *Uddhyana Bandha* (diaphragm lock). Repeat for 1–3 minutes.

The abdomen is the central point of your power and sovereignty. Uddhyana Bandha works the digestive organs and heart.

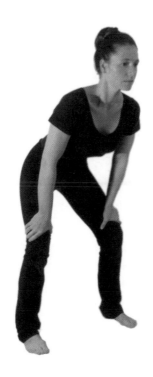

b) Place your feet hip-width apart and your hands on your hips. Pull up your pelvic floor and then make large circles with your upper body. Every time you come to the front, change direction. Breathe in as your upper body starts to come forwards and breathe out as your upper body starts to go backwards. 2 minutes.

The hips symbolise perseverance, and so your ability to stay the course is strengthened through this exercise.

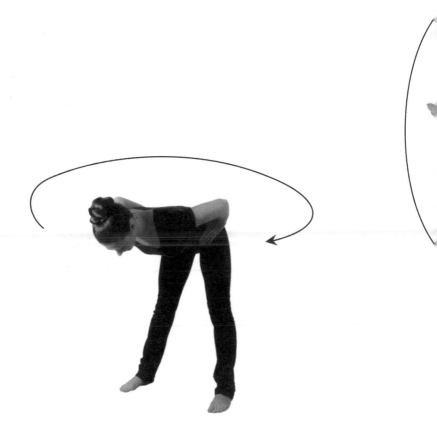

c) Place your feet hip-width apart and stretch your arms out to your sides. At the same time as breathing out and bending forwards from your hips with a straight back, swing your arms forwards eight times making large circles. Now change the direction of your circles, and as you breathe in, slowly bring yourself upright again. 4–5 minutes.

The arm meridians flow straight into the brain; because of this, this type of movement integrates the two halves of the brain. This exercise also helps to prevent arthritis and rejuvenates the spine.

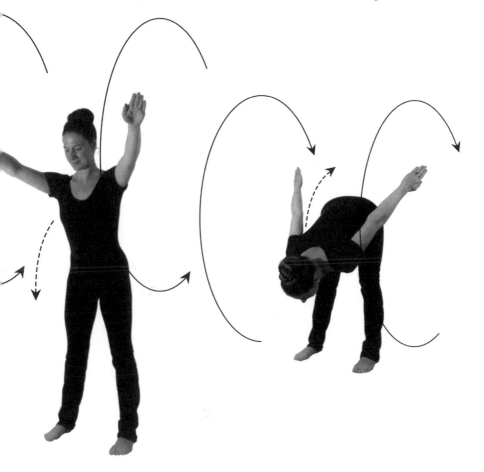

Grace, Part 2

a) Place your feet about 50 cm apart; tighten your pelvic floor and as you breathe in, stretch your arms high over your head and then slowly lift your chin and stretch your neck. As you breathe out, let yourself go forwards, bending at the hips until your palms are flat on the floor. 2 minutes.

This exercise wakes up your whole system, and the different parts of you begin to function as a whole.

See how it goes, your hands may not reach the floor. You can put them on your thighs instead.

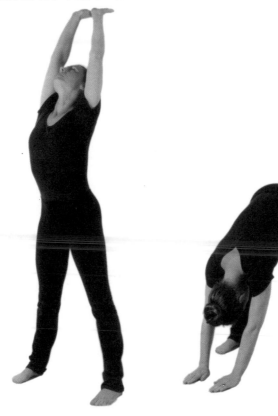

b) Spread your legs so that your feet are about 90 cm apart. Keep your pelvic floor pulled up. As you breathe in, stretch your arms over your head, lifting up your chin, and pushing up with your wrists. As you breathe out, bend to the front keeping your back straight and your pelvic floor contracted. Keep going until your palms make contact with the ground. 1 minute.

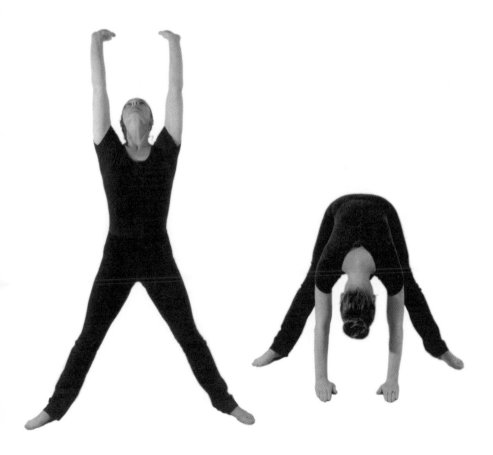

c) Put your feet together. Keep your pelvic floor pulled up as you breathe in and stretch your arms over your head, pushing up your chin. As you breathe out, bend to the front, keeping your back straight and your pelvic floor contracted. Keep going until your palms make contact with the ground. 1minute.

This is a balancing exercise. It will help your staying power, and has a positive effect on the lymphatic system.

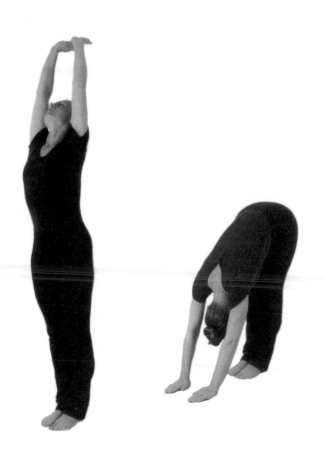

Grace, Part 3

a) The Archer. Put your right foot about 75 cm in front of your left foot. Your left foot is pointing outwards at about a 45-degree angle. Put most of your weight on the front foot and stretch out your back leg. Your hips should point to the front. Hold your right arm in front of you and make a fist with your right hand whilst holding up your thumb. The general feeling is that you are holding a bow. Make a fist with your left arm too, bringing it back to your left shoulder. Stretch your left elbow backwards at shoulder height, as if you were about to loose an arrow from the bow. As you breathe out, bend your front knee; as you breathe in, bring it back to your starting position. Keep your eyes focused on the tip of your thumb. After 1–3 minutes, change sides.

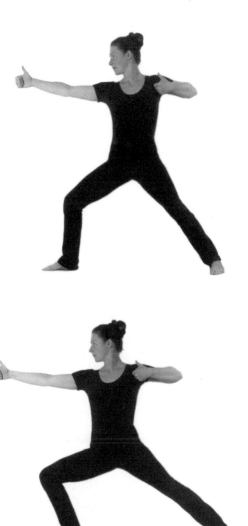

This exercise builds your inner strength and your ability to calmly pursue and reach your goals. It also works on the heart and sexual energy. If you need to, just make small movements with your leading knee.

b) Place your feet hip-width apart. Now put your hands on your shoulders, with your fingers pointing to your neck. As you breathe in, push your arms up; and as you breathe out, bring them back to your shoulders again. Do this movement extremely quickly, whilst breathing powerfully from your abdomen. 30 seconds.

This exercise lifts energy to your crown chakra, which is called the Sahasrara or lotus of a thousand petals. It will give you the feeling of being at one.

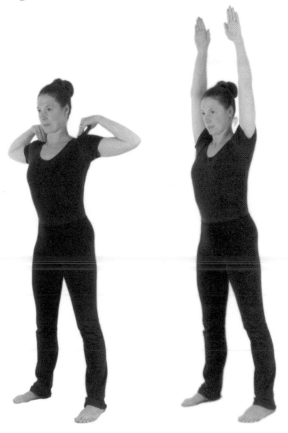

c) Bring your heels together and spread out your toes. Stretch your arms high above your head, fingers interlocked and palms facing upwards. Keep your eyes shut. Do the Breath of Fire for 1–3 minutes.

For directions on the Breath of Fire see p. 47

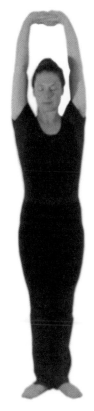

Relaxation
(standing, sitting or lying) 1–11 minutes
Listen to the whispering of the leaves and branches, and the stillness that surrounds everything.

Meditation for inner strength

(YB 10 Jan. 1978)

Sit in an easy posture with your legs crossed and your spine straight. Bring your hands together into the prayer Mudra, crossing your right thumb over your left thumb. Press the base of your thumbs against your breastbone at heart level.

Let your breath flow freely and calmly. Have your eyes just 1/10 open and direct your gaze to the tip of your nose. Dive deeply into the highest level of being. Melt into your higher self, and allow a feeling of utter simplicity to exist in your centre, letting go of all expectation.

Try to relax your spirit and calm your intellect, so that your thoughts quieten.

Start with 11 minutes and then gradually increase to 31 minutes.

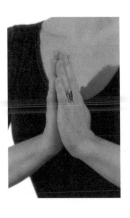
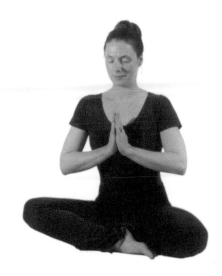

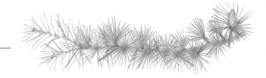

This meditation neutralises negativity, and is comforting and centring. It enables you to enter into the reality of your godhead.

The prayer Mudra neutralises negativity and energetically integrates your body by bringing together left and right.

ELDER

(Sambucus nigra)

Every species of tree effects the landscape that it is part of, and the human soul too. The tree's power to do this, however, is not necessarily determined by its physical size. The modest appearance of the elder is a great example of this. Being small and generally multi-stemmed, it looks more like a bush than a tree. Yet its legend is remarkable. It appears in more myths, stories and folktales than some of the 'great' trees that dominate the landscape.

Elder and lime are the only two European trees from which every part can be used to heal the human being. Because of the pressure that human overpopulation puts on trees, we don't want to recommend that you go out and use the bark, roots or too many leaves of this wonderful tree, but we can highly recommend both flowers and berries to you. Elderflowers break fevers, and are generally calming for the human organism. (For treating a cold, make a tea with 1–2 teaspoons of the flowers in a cup, pour freshly boiled water over them, cover and leave for 5 minutes before drinking.) The berries ripen in early autumn and are great preventative medicine. They are loaded with vitamins and strengthen the immune system. The best way of taking them is as juice. Boil them up for a few minutes, press them and then strain the juice, which you can then drink hot with honey. You could always make concentrate or jam from them, too. In prehistoric times the elder was connected to important goddesses. Northern European folklore associates this tree with the compassionate, nourishing and healing side of the earth spirits. It was traditional for farmers to plant an elder tree near the house as the sacred dwelling of the house spirit. Well into the middle of the 19th century, weekly offerings were made to this tree, mostly milk, cake or bread.

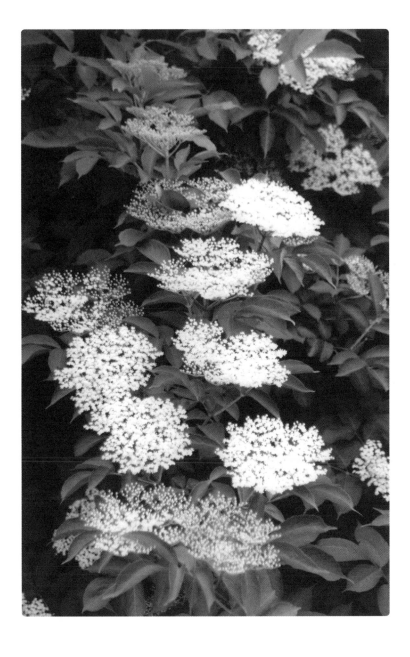

In German-speaking countries it was common, until the beginning of the 20th century, to see people taking their hats off to the elder tree as they walked past. Before the tendencies of mainly patriarchal religions to place greater importance on male deities, goddesses were seen as the source of all life. The mother of the universe in her smaller form was the earth mother. Before creation, she contained within herself the potential of all life, first giving birth to the male principle, often in primeval times depicted as a serpent. On the earthly plane, depending on the tradition, this energy is either symbolised as the Green man, sky-god, weather-god, or lord of the dance. Together they are the divine couple that bring forth all living things.

A ritual song, first written down in Russia in the 19th century, connects the elder with the primeval forces of creation.

The old Elder trees sing –
They sing of life, they sing of death,
They sing of the whole human race.
The old Elders bestow
Long life on the whole earth;
But to the other, the bad death,
The old Elders command
A long and far journey.
The old Elders promise
Eternal life
To the whole of Humankind.

The key words that attune us to the spiritual world of the elder tree are *abundance, spiritual nourishment, trust* and *gratitude.*

Exercise Sequence for Abundance

We recommend that you carry out these exercises either under or in view of an elder tree. If that's not possible, you can visualise an elder. The energy of the tree strengthens the effect of the exercises.

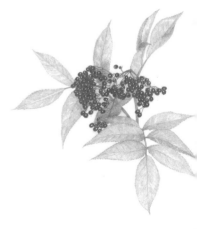

Abundance, Part 1

a) Tree pose. Stand on your right leg and bring your left foot to your groin or on the inside of your right thigh. Stretch your arms high above your head, palms together. Focus on one spot at eye level and breathe long and deep. 1–3 minutes, then change sides.

Strengthens the large muscles that run up either side of your back and has a grounding effect. If you need help balancing yourself, rest one hand on the tree, or on a wall.

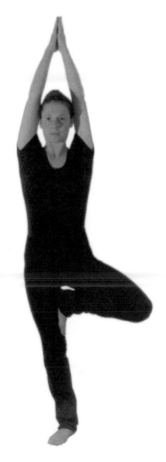

b) Place your feet hip-width apart, lift up your arms so that they are 60 degrees apart with elbows straight. As you breathe in, turn your whole body to the left; and then as you breathe out, turn to the right. With your eyes shut, direct both eyes to your third eye. Perform quick turns for 1–3 minutes.

Works the liver and develops trust.

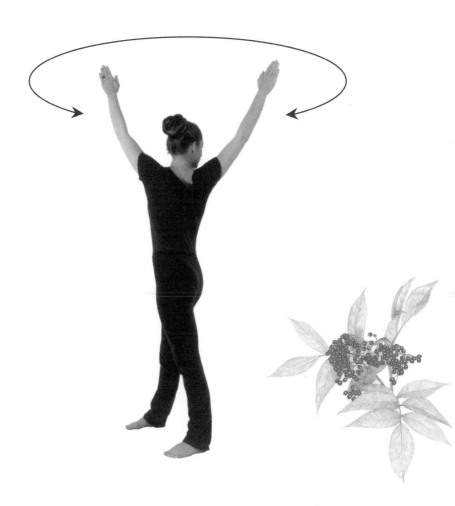

c) Place your feet hip-width apart, hands on your hips. Bend your upper body forwards from your hips, keeping your back straight and your head up. Direct your gaze forwards. Breathe long and deep for 1–3 minutes.

Corrects spinal imbalances.

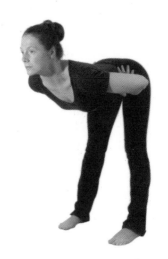

Abundance, Part 2

a) Place your feet hip-width apart and close your eyes. Breathe in and open your eyes, purse your lips, and sink your head so that your chin touches your breastbone. Now breathe out, close your eyes, blow out your cheeks and slowly bring your head up again. Repeat for 1–2 minutes.

Relaxes the facial muscles and increases the flow of blood to the face.

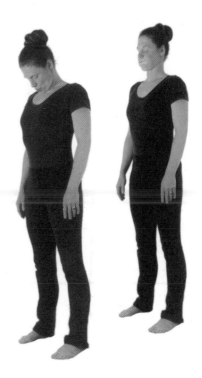

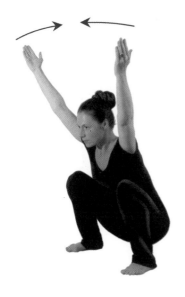

b) Adopt the crouching pose and stretch your arms up so that they are about 60 degrees apart. With powerful movements, clap your hands. 30 seconds.

Wakes up the spirit and harmonises the nervous system.

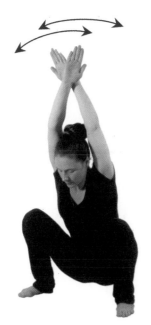

c) Maintain the same pose and make a scissoring movement with your arms, without letting them touch one another. As you bring them apart, breathe in and as they cross one another breathe out. 2 minutes 30 seconds.

d) Stand up again, place your feet hip-width apart, and focus on a point about 1.5 metres in front of your toes, or stand 1.5 metres from the tree and focus on the base of its trunk. Do Breath of Fire. 1–3 minutes.

This anchors your trust in a positive future.
Try not to blink.

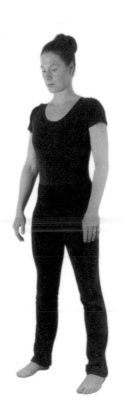

Abundance, Part 3

The Archer

Put your right foot about 75 cm in front of your left foot. Your left foot is pointing outwards at about a 45-degree angle. Put most of your weight on the front foot and stretch out your back leg. Your hips should point to the front. Hold your right arm in front of you and make a fist with your right hand whilst holding up your thumb. The general feeling is one of holding a bow. Make a fist with your left arm too, bringing it back to your left shoulder. Stretch your left elbow backwards at shoulder height, as if you were about to loose an arrow from the bow. Keep your eyes focused on the tip of your thumb. After 1–3 minutes, change sides. Now you can follow the steps below.

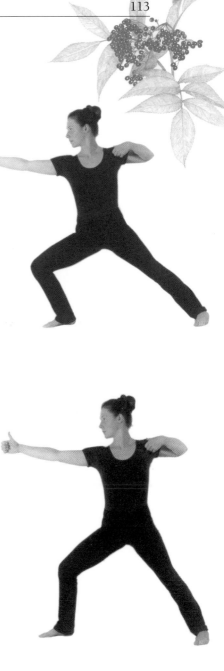

a) Bend your front knee so that it comes over your big toe, four times, each time coming back to the starting position. Do this whilst singing SA TA NA MA. One bend of the knee should last about 1 second. Sing one syllable per bend.

b) Now, keeping your feet in the same place, bend your knee again with your hands placed either side of your right foot, singing SA TA NA MA again, one syllable per movement, just like last time.

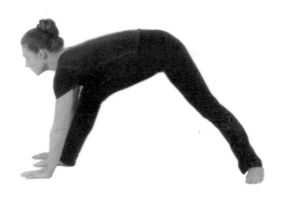

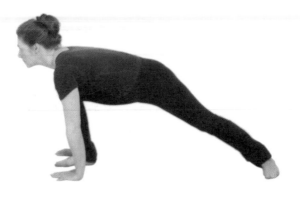

c) Still with the same movement of the knee, and feet in the same position, stretch your arms above your head, palms facing upwards. Sing SA TA NA MA, one syllable to accompany each of the four movements.

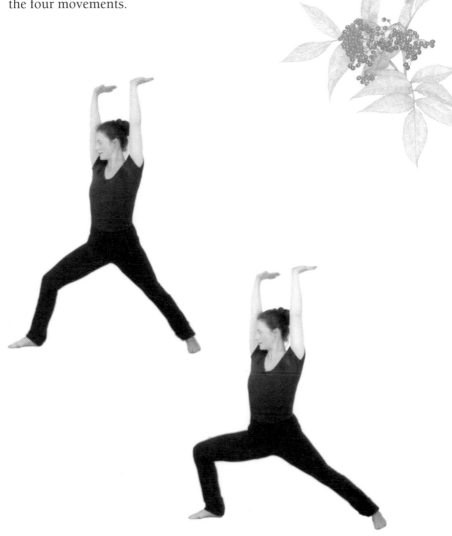

d) Still with the same movement of the knee, and feet in the same position, with outstretched arms clap above your head while singing SA TA NA MA again.

Go through the sequence a) to d) for five minutes, before changing legs and doing it again, but this time for only 3 minutes.

Strengthens your confidence and ability to set goals and achieve them. SA translates as eternity or birth, TA means life, NA means death, and MA is new beginning.

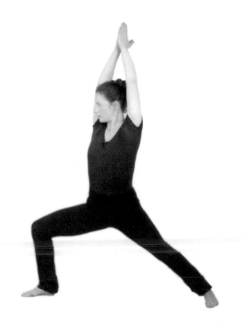

Relaxation
(standing, sitting or lying down) 1–11 minutes
Listen to the whispering of the leaves and branches, and the stillness that surrounds everything.

Meditation for Gratitude

(YB 1 May 1978)

Sit cross-legged holding your hands in the shape of a bowl in front of your heart chakra, so that you can collect sacred blessings known as *Gurprasaad*. At first have your eyes 1/10 open, your gaze directed to the end of your nose, then as you meditate gradually allow them to close.

Become completely still. Know that you are a part of creation. Let your hands fill up with everything that you need to become happy.

You can decide yourself how long to meditate for.

Yogi Bhajan said; 'Count your blessings not your problems.'

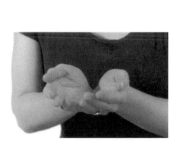
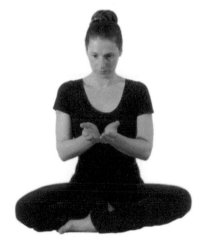

LIME
(Tilia)

The lime is the tree of healing. According to herbal lore, no plant in Europe has such a broad spectrum of medicinal uses. Its leaves, flowers, bark and roots have long been used, and still are, to promote human well-being. Early on, the lime was honoured with a place in Greek mythology because of its many gifts to humanity. Asklepius, founder of western medicine, gained his wisdom from the centaur Chiron, son of Phylira. Phylira is the original spirit of the lime.

For many Anglo-Saxon and other Germanic peoples, the most sacred tribal centre was an old lime tree. At that time, the lime was attributed with radiating godly wisdom, truth, justice and clarity. It was here also that people found a balance between empathy and will. The lime was sacred to Freyja, goddess of earth and love.

During Christian-dominated times, the sacred lime transformed into the customary village lime, a place for meetings and gatherings. Well into the 19th century, the lime was protector of the home in Scandinavian lore.

The old English and German word for lime is *linden*, from *lindern*, which means *to alleviate* or *to provide relief*. But there is another hidden side to this tree. Northern legends tell how Sigurd slayed a dragon in an attempt to use its blood to become invincible, but his plan was thwarted because a leaf from a lime tree fell unnoticed on his shoulder. It is interesting that the dragons lair must therefore have been close to a lime tree or grove, making the lime, giver of peace, relief and healing, the guardian of the fiery and wild life-force that lies beneath the earth's crust. This is

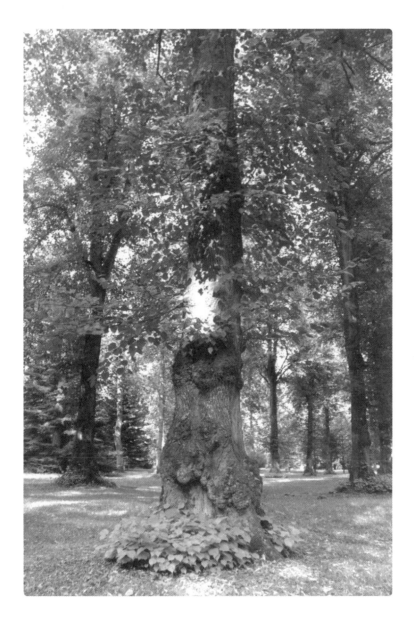

also indicated by the German word *linden,* which is related to the ancient word for dragon: *lindworm.*

Sigurd's ridiculous plan to become invincible by bathing in dragon's blood was obviously contrary to his code of honour as a spiritual warrior. Seen in this way, the lime was working with his higher self to prevent him from making a big mistake.

> The key words to attune us to the spirit of the lime tree are *balance, healing, peace* and *tolerance.*

Healing Exercise Sequence

We recommend that you carry out these exercises either under or in view of a lime tree. If that's not possible, you can visualise a lime tree. The energy of the tree strengthens the effect of the exercises.

Healing, Part 1

a) Place your feet hip-width apart and stretch your arms straight up. As you breathe in, bend to the left, stretching your right side; as you breathe out, bend to your right. 26 times for each side.

This exercise stretches your rib muscles and activates the lymphatic system.

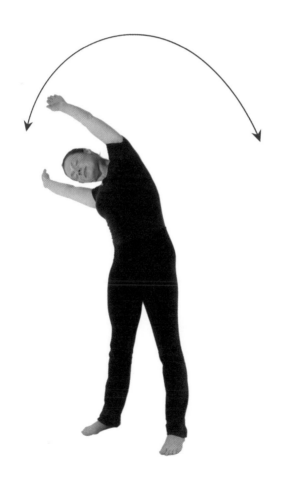

b) Stretch your legs about 60 cm apart. Tighten your pelvic floor and bend your upper body forwards. Stretch your arms between your legs so that your hands are pointing backwards, palms down as if you wanted to touch the ground behind you. As you breathe deeply, hold this position. 1 minute. Staying in this position, now make a u-shape with your tongue and stick it out of your mouth. Now do the Breath of Fire through your rolled tongue. 1 minute.

This is a cleansing exercise for the liver and benefits blood circulation to the head.

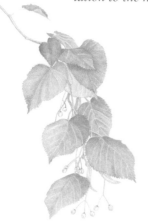

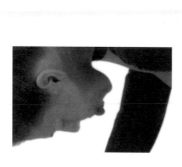

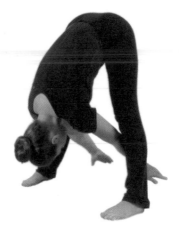

c) Again spread your legs about 60 cm apart, and put your right hand on your hip while your left hand goes on your back, up between your shoulder blades. Breathe in as you turn to the left. Keep your eyes shut and your gaze inwardly directed to your third eye. 1–3 minutes. (One side only.)

This exercise is good for the heart.

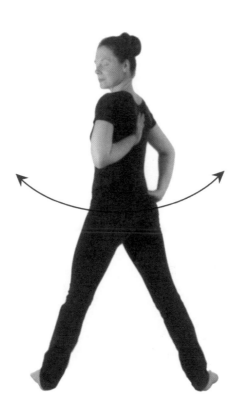

Healing, Part 2

a) Chair pose.

Place your feet a little further than hip-width apart. Keeping your back straight, bend your knees and bring your forearms down to your calves until you are clutching your ankles with your hands. Elevate your head and focus your gaze on a point on the lime tree or on a nearby wall. Breathe long and slow. 1–3 minutes.

The chair pose cleans the blood.

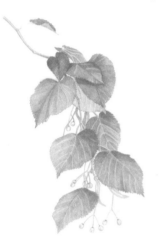

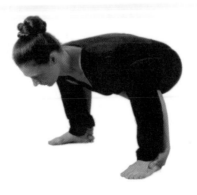

b) Spread your feet about 90 cm apart and put your hands on your hips. Breathe in and turn your upper-body and head to the left. As you breathe out, turn to your right. Keep your eyes shut and your inner gaze focused on your third eye. 1–3 minutes.

This exercise stimulates self-healing.

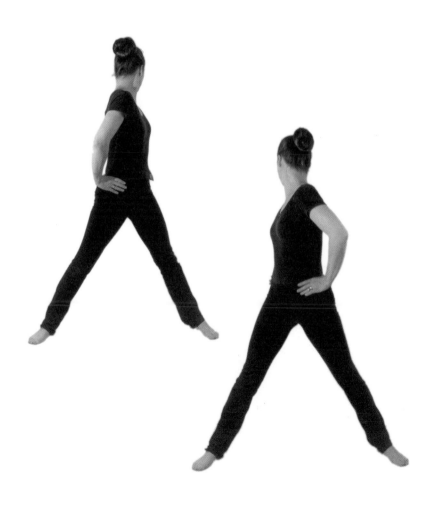

c) Again with your feet spread, hold out your arms horizontally. Tighten your pelvic floor, taking your left hand to your right foot, while at the same time holding your right hand up straight up and looking at your right hand. Stay as you are and do the Breath of Fire. 1–3 minutes.

Then breathe in deeply; before breathing out and with your pelvic floor engaged, bring yourself to standing again. Change sides and fire breathe once more. 1–3 minutes.

This exercise integrates the body and the two hemispheres of the brain.

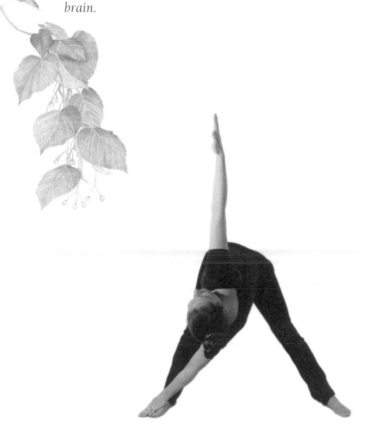

Healing, Part 3

a) The 'Yogi Twist'.

Place your feet hip-width apart, and then bring your elbows up to shoulder height, your forearms vertical. Turn your palms forwards, fingers in the *Gyan Mudra* (forefinger and thumb together). Lift your chest; stretch your neck; and as you breathe in, turn your upper body to the left, and then to the right as you breathe out. Your feet need to stay flat on the floor. Keep your spine vertical and close your eyes, with your inner gaze directed to your third eye. 1–11 minutes.

This movement is very beneficial for the liver.

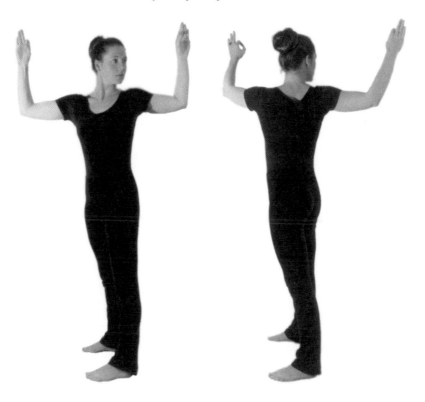

b) Bring your feet together so that they are touching. Stretch out your arms to the sides at shoulder height. As you breathe in, bend your upper body to the left, stretching your right arm up to heaven. As you breathe out, bend down to your right and stretch up your left arm. Keep your arms in one line.

This exercise regulates the functioning of your thoracic vertebra.

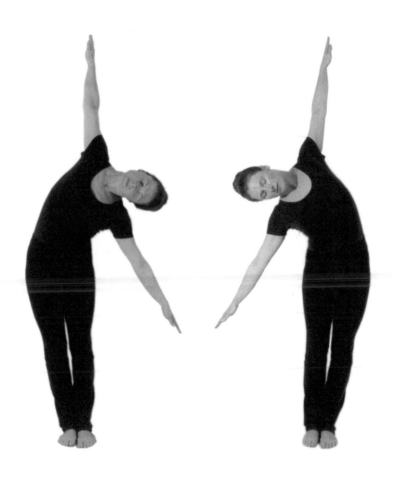

c) Keeping your feet together, stretch your legs and pull your coccyx in a little. Tighten your pelvic floor and lift your arms way up high over your head. Bring your palms together. Lift your chest, and stretch up and back as far as you can. Close your eyes and do the Breath of Fire. 1–3 minutes.

Now breathe in deeply, breathe out again and bring yourself upright, back to the starting position. Then let your upper body hang down to the front. 1 minute.

This exercise strengthens the functioning of the lungs.

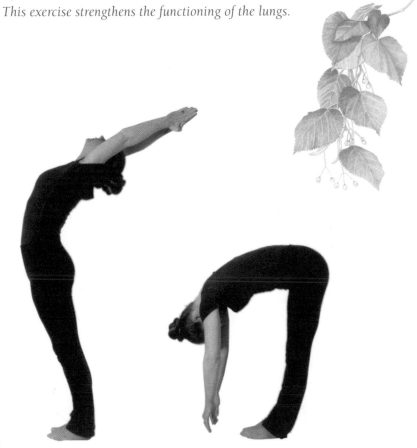

Relaxation
(standing, sitting or lying) 1–11 minutes
Listen to the whispering of the leaves and branches, and the stillness that surrounds everything.

Healing meditation
For the tree, for you and for others.
Sing:

Ra Ma Da Sa Sa Se So Hong

Use different Mudras depending on what you want to use the healing meditation for:

Distant healing Mudra: Support your elbows on your ribs, hold your forearms angled upwards in front of you, and turn your palms outwards with your fingers close together; keep your fingers straight and pointing downwards.

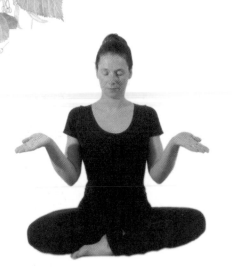 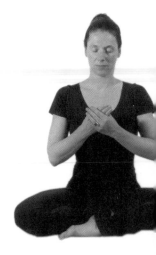

Self healing Mudra: Put the back of your right hand in your left palm, with your right thumb over your left thumb. Hold your hands about 30 cm away from your heart.

Healing Mudra for healing someone who is there with you: Stretch out your arms with about 60 degrees between them, palms facing forwards. 11 minutes.

To end the meditation:
Breathe in, hold your breath, and visualise a connection between your heart and your hands. Then, breathe out and visualise this energy flowing out of your hands.

Choose your own rhythm and tune to accompany this mantra.

To hear a traditional tune, go to Satya's website:
www.satyasingh.com/treeyoga

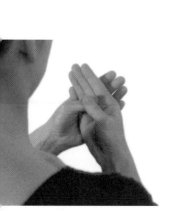

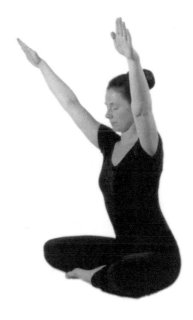

PINE
(Pinus)

The pine is one of the pioneer trees, and is more than deserving of the name. Pioneer trees give us the strength to venture out into the unknown and establish ourselves outside our comfort zone. To do this we have to trust our new situation enough to send out roots, and establish ourselves with serious determination. The individualistic approach of the pine tree also shows in the way it grows – there's lots of room for variety. While most European coniferous trees, especially fir and spruce, usually exhibit a geometrical, cone-like shape, pine doesn't even grow particularly symmetrically in thick woodland. A single pine is often a very striking, storm-torn being with a strong personality.

All plants and especially trees display a remarkable degree of flexibility, but it is the pine that stands out head and shoulders above the rest in this regard. Within temperate regions they can thrive on damp moorland, as well as on very poor soils, cliff-faces, and even sand. It's very common to see a group of them standing by the sea on the edge of a sand dune, withstanding the salt-laden winds that buffet their crowns. Some members of the pine family can survive extreme and lengthy periods of cold weather, living in mountainous regions or enduring Scandinavian winters, while others thrive in parched soils under the baking Mediterranean sun.

Since records began, pines have been held in esteem for their great strength. An example of this is that pine is by far the most widespread tree among the traditional Scottish clan badges.

According to one of the oldest religious cults of Europe and the Near East, the pine is the dwelling place of the god of plant life himself, the Anatolian Attis. In world mythology the spirit of

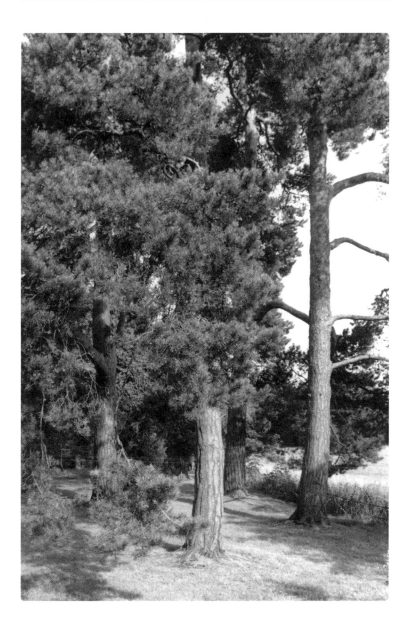

plant life is usually portrayed as some sort of Green Man, son of the great nature goddess. These myths speak of the annual growth and hibernation cycle of plants as mirroring the cyclic death and re-birth of the god of fertility. In the myth of Attis and Kybele, which was developed in Anatolia and then spread to Greece and Italy, Kybele is the great mother and Attis her son. He dies after having castrated himself, and is transformed into a pine tree. Hence the vital role the pine played in the rituals of this culture.

Myths describe inner events through the symbolic use of external events. The wisdom of the Attis myth does not lie in self-mutilation, but in the necessity that we direct and channel our sexual and creative energy.

> The key words that attune us to the spiritual realm of the pine are *self-discipline*, *endurance*, *courage* and *grace*.

Exercise Sequence for Building Courage

We recommend that you carry out these exercises either under or in view of a pine tree. If that's not possible, you can visualise a pine. The energy of the tree strengthens the effect of the exercises.

Courage, Part 1

a) Jog on the spot. While you are doing this, cross your arms in front of your chest if you are a woman; or if you are a man, bring your elbows up by your sides to the height of your shoulders, with your forearms hanging down vertically. Your hands are in the *Gyan Mudra*. Breathe rhythmically; for example, take four steps as you breathe in and four as you breathe out. Tighten your pelvic floor as you exercise. 5 minutes.

Cleanses the blood.

Of course you can turn this into a jog through the woodland if that is where you are.

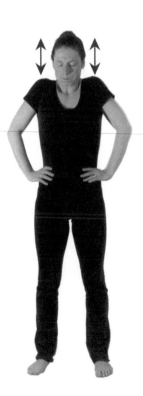

b) Put your hands on your hips. Close your eyes. Breathe in and blow out your cheeks. Hold your breath and as you do so, powerfully move your shoulders up and down a number of times. Then while you breathe out, relax your cheeks and shoulders. Repeat this cycle for 1 minute.

Relaxes the face and strengthens the lymphatic system.

c) Place your feet hip-width apart; bring your elbows to the front and up to shoulder height with your forearms pointing upwards at 90 degrees to your arms. Make a fist, enclosing your thumbs with your fingers. Breathe in and take your elbows out to your sides and your forearms parallel to the floor at the same angle as before; now breathe out and bring your elbows back to the front and your starting position. Repeat for 1–3 minutes.

Strengthens the shoulders and lungs.

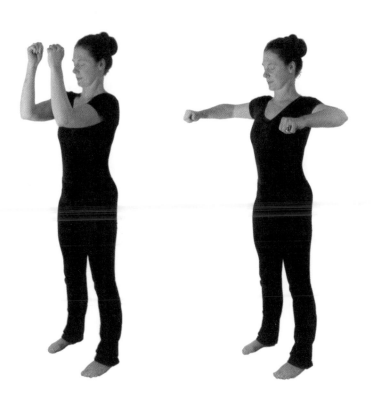

Courage, Part 2

a) Place your feet as far apart as you can. Bring your forearms up in front of your body, parallel to the ground, and let your hands hang loose. As you breathe in, circle forwards with your hips; and as you breathe out, circle backwards. Choose one direction and keep going for 2 minutes.

This exercise strengthens your warrior spirit and can also be done separately from the rest of the sequence. Legend has it that Moses made his people do this exercise to prepare them for trouble and give them an unbending will in the face of conflict.

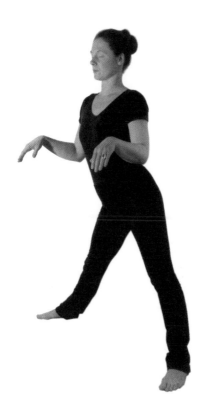

b) Place your feet hip-width apart; interlace your fingers, palms touching in the Venus grip, then tighten your pelvic floor, and as you breathe in lift your chest and stretch your arms up and behind you. As you breathe out, bend both your upper body and your arms forwards. Make these movements fluid and swift. 4 minutes.

Enlivens the circulation and strengthens the lungs.

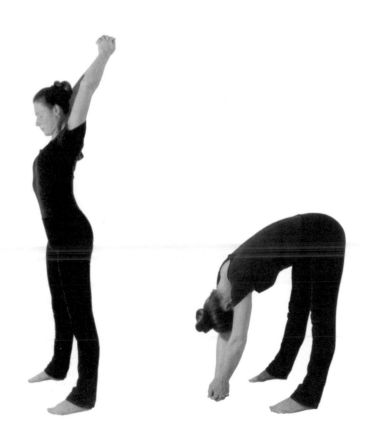

c) Stretch your arms high above your head, clasp your fingers together, and turn your palms upwards. Without lifting your feet from the ground, shake your legs intensively for one minute. Now shake your whole body for a further minute at the same time as using the tip of your tongue to repeat the *mantra* 'HAR'.

This exercise clears blocks in the legs and back. HAR means 'God in you'. If you roll your r's your tongue will stimulate the reflex area to your brain, which is on the inside of the roof of your mouth.

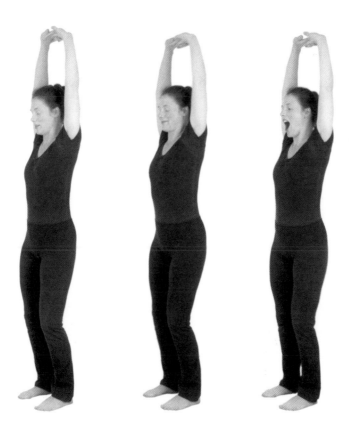

Courage, Part 3

The Archer

Put your right foot about 75 cm in front of your left foot. Your left foot is pointing outwards at about a 45-degree angle. Put most of your weight on the front foot and stretch out your back leg. Your hips should point to the front. Hold your right arm in front of you and make a fist with your right hand whilst holding up your thumb. The general feeling is one of holding a bow. Make a fist with your left arm too, bringing it back to your left shoulder. Stretch your left elbow backwards at shoulder height, as if you were about to loose an arrow from the bow. Keep your eyes focused on the tip of your thumb. After 1–3 minutes, change sides. Now you can follow the steps below:

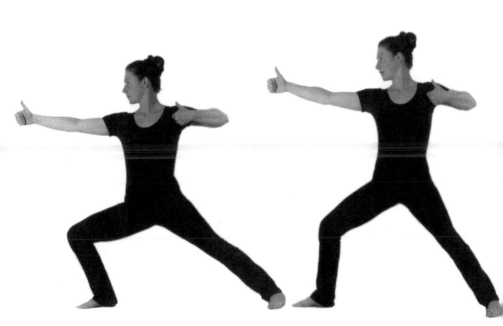

a) Bend your front knee so that it comes over your big toe, four times, each time coming back to the starting position. Do this whilst singing SA TA NA MA. One bend of the knee should last about 1 second. Sing one syllable per bend.

b) Now, keeping your feet in the same place, bend your knee again, once per syllable, clapping your hands above your head, singing SA TA NA MA again, one syllable per movement, just like last time.

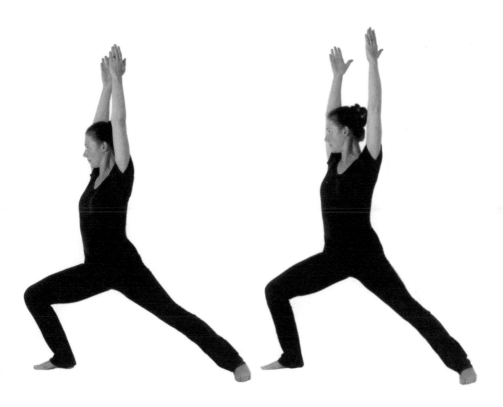

c) Still with the same movement of the knee, and feet in the same position, stretch your arms in front of you clapping your hands. Sing SA TA NA MA, four movements to accompany each syllable.

d) Still with the same movement, feet in the same position, clap behind your back while singing SA TA NA MA. Four times per syllable.

Go through the sequence a) to d) for five minutes, before changing legs and doing it again for 5 minutes. The whole time you are doing the Archer pose, focus on one point on the pine tree, or nearby wall, without blinking.

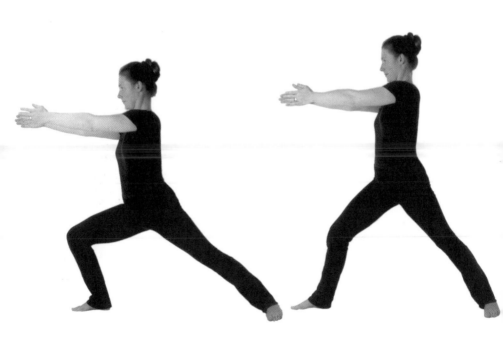

You can bend your knees really gently, and certainly bend it no further than over your big toe.

The Archer is the best pose to teach you to be able to set your sights on something and achieve your goal. It brings clarity and concentration, strengthens the nerves and digestion, and cleanses the body of poisons. The Archer has a positive effect on all 108 minerals of the body, particularly on the calcium, magnesium and calcium balance. Regular practice prevents deficiencies of these minerals.

SA translates as eternity or birth, TA means life, NA means death, and MA stands for new beginning. If you want to hear the tune go to: *www.satyasingh.com/treeyoga*

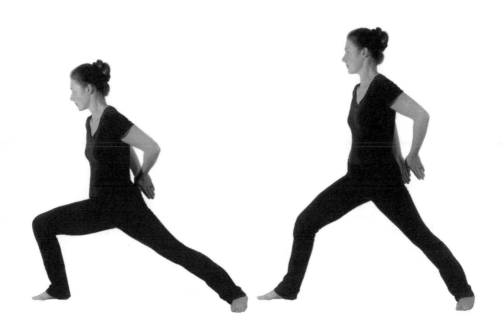

Relaxation
(standing, sitting, or lying) 1–11 minutes
Listen the rustling of the leaves, and the stillness that surrounds
everything.

Meditation on sacred law

(YB 6 Jan. 1977)

Easy Pose

Sit cross legged and bend back your left hand so that your palm faces upwards and your fingers point to the left. The top of your palms should be a couple of centimetres under your chin. Your left forearm is vertical and in front of your chest.

Bring your right forearm between your body and your left forearm, putting the palm of your right hand under your left hand. Grasp the outside of your left hand firmly. Breathe long and deep. Keep your eyes 1/10 open. In your thoughts repeat a mantra that you like. Start with 11 minutes and then gradually increase to 31 minutes.

When you have finished, stay sitting still for a while, close your eyes and feel well.

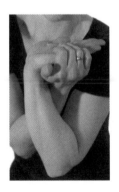
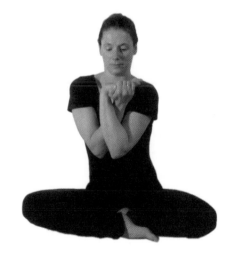

ROWAN

(Sorbus aucuparia)

Rowan belongs to the rose family, and is a fruiting tree found in cooler, temperate regions. Its bitter red berries are not poisonous, yet if eaten raw they can irritate the stomach lining. The parasorbic acid that causes this irritation can be rendered harmless by cooking the berries gently, which will also preserve most of their vitamin content. Rowan berries contain more vitamin C than citrus fruits.

Despite its quite modest size, the rowan was once one of the most worshipped trees in the northern hemisphere, from Ireland to Russia. And, wherever we look, we see it has been used for protection. Countless invocations include this tree, and it was used to make talismans and good luck charms. There is an Icelandic myth in which even Thor the mighty thunder god has his life saved by a rowan tree. But it is Celtic wisdom that most clearly elucidates the meaning of this tree. According to Druidic lore the rowan is the tree of the bard, and its gift to the world is *Awen*, true inspiration. Inspiration is our alternative to following dogma, and attunes our consciousness to the deeper truths.

The ancient Celtic bards travelled the land, keeping the myths and legends alive in people's minds. The function of myths and legends is to explain the origins of things, to show our roots to us and how we fit into the all-encompassing web of life. Hence the bardic tradition was psychologically, socially and energetically responsible for maintaining harmony between human and environment. So we see the intimate connection that exists between protection and inspiration.

In this way the rowan has inspired us in the creation of this book. *Tree Yoga* is just as Druidic a book as it is Yogic: it is about

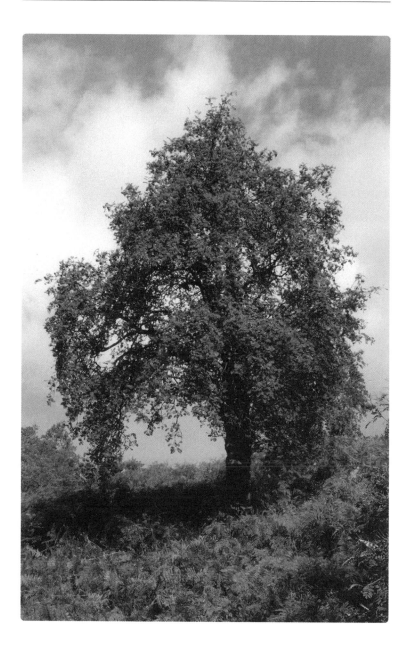

the healing and growth of each of us as individuals, acting in harmony with all living beings.

> The key words to attune yourself with the spiritual realm of the rowan are *inspiration*, *the voice of the heart*, and *protection*.

Exercise Sequence for Inspiration

We recommend that you carry out these exercises either under or in view of a rowan tree. If that's not possible you can visualise a rowan. The energy of the tree strengthens the effect of the exercise.

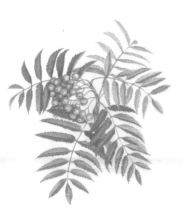

Inspiration, Part 1

a) Place your feet about 15 cm apart. Feel the soles of your feet in contact with the ground. Bend your knees a little, and let your pelvis rotate slowly. Feel how your pelvis is connected to your knees and feet. Then slowly circle your upper body, shoulders and head. Now bring your hands above your head and comb through your aura from above to below with lightly stretched fingers. Take your hands all through your aura with a cleansing action. 1–3 minutes.

This exercise enhances the ability of the Auric and magnetic fields to act as energetic filters.

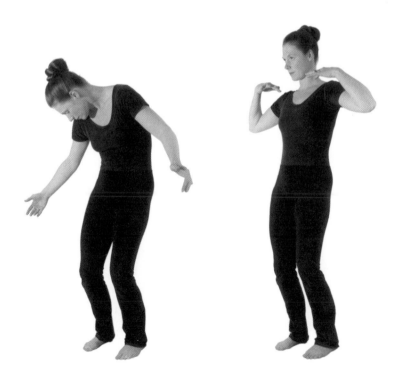

b) Breathe in, hold your breath, tighten your anal sphincter and pull it upwards, then breathe out and relax it. Repeat for 1 minute.

c) Breathe in, hold your breath and pull in your anus again, this time also tightening and pulling up the muscles around your genitalia. Then breathe out and relax. Repeat for 1 minute.

Pelvic floor exercises stimulate your organs, breath, voice, and improve your posture.

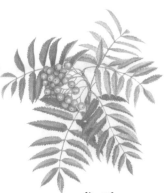

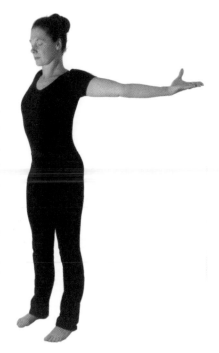

d) Place your feet hip-width apart. Stretch out your arms to your sides with your palms facing upwards, pulling your arms backwards slightly. Your fingers are stretched out horizontally, your thumbs pointing upwards. Close your eyes and do the Breath of Fire while holding this pose for 2 minutes.

Then slowly bring your arms over your head until your thumbs meet. Tense your pelvic floor, lift your chest and stretch your body backwards in the form of a bow. To finish the exercise, breathe out, bend your body forwards and then touch your toes.

This exercise energises your electromagnetic field.

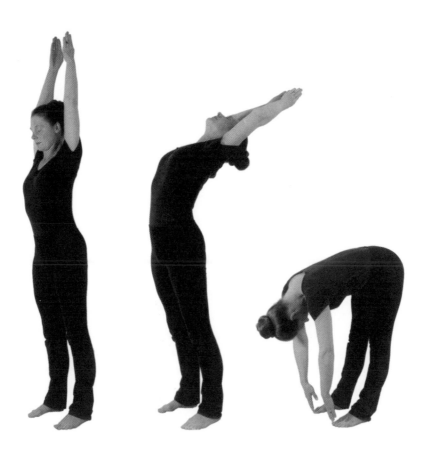

Inspiration, Part 2

a) Place your feet between 60 and 90 cm apart. Keep them flat on the floor as you bend your knees until your thighs are parallel to the ground, as if you were sitting on a stool. Also hold your forearms parallel to the ground, palms down, and gently bend forwards. Holding this pose, bob up as you breathe in and down as you breathe out, also bouncing to the left and right. Keep your eyes shut and sense your energy field. 2–3 minutes.

This godsend of an exercise connects us to the earth.

You can crouch down a little less, keeping your backside higher than your knees if they are weak.

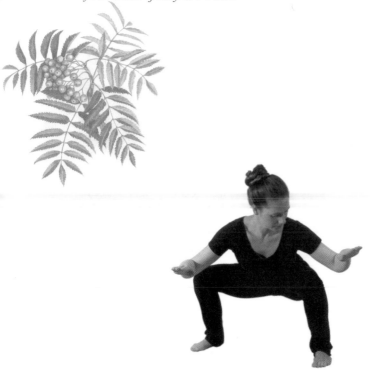

b) Kundalini Pran Dandh

Stand up again and put your weight on your left leg. Lift up your right leg so that it is horizontal and pointing in front of you. With both hands, hold on to your right ankle or calf. Keep both legs stretched. Find a point on the rowan tree or a nearby wall and focus on it. Breathe long and deep. After 2–3 minutes, change sides and repeat the pose with your left leg in the air, again for 2–3 minutes.

Kundalini Pran Dandh means Kundalini energy rod. This exercise strengthens the heart and aura. You can support yourself on the tree or wall if you need to.

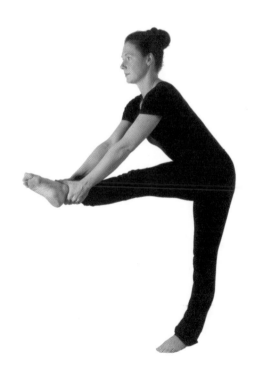

c) Place your feet about 30 cm apart. Fold your fingers together in the Venus grip, pointing with both forefingers stretched out. Your right thumb is underneath your left thumb. Keep your pelvic floor engaged and stretch your arms high over your head. As you breathe out, bend forwards until your forefingers touch the ground. Swing round to your left, and as you breathe in stand upright again, with your arms held high above your head. As you breathe out bend down straight in front of you, and then with your in-breath stand straight up again. Then as you breathe out bend down again, swing around to your left, and then as you breathe in stand up again. Do this sequence for 2 minutes.

This exercise causes the energy in
your aura to flow.

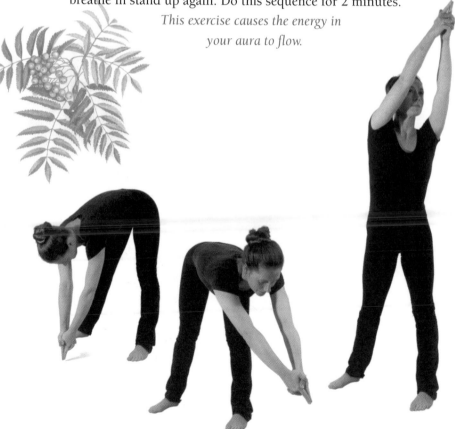

Inspiration, Part 3

a) Place your feet hip-width apart. Stretch your arms out to the sides at shoulder height, with your fingers pointing straight and pressed gently together, palms facing downwards. Now, as you breathe out let your arms sink about 20 cm, and then as you breathe in bring them back up to the starting position. Then as you breathe out lift them by about 20 cm, again bringing them back again as you breathe in. Do this exercise at a comfortable speed. Put equal emphasis on your out-breath and in-breath. 1–3 minutes.

This exercise integrates the two hemispheres of the brain and strengthens the nervous system.

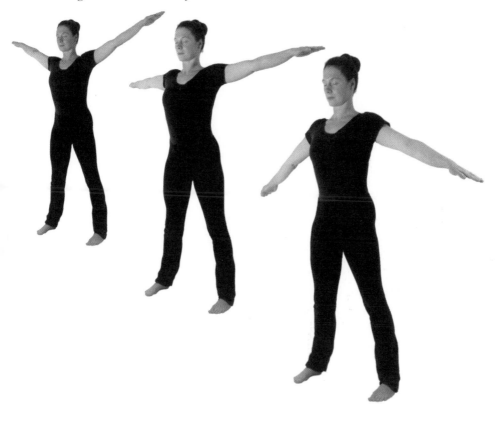

b) Stand in a relaxed and upright posture and concentrate on your third eye (in the centre between your eyebrows). Also direct your eyes, while shut, towards this point. Imagine that you are breathing in and out from where the bridge of your nose meets your face, and place your attention on what that feels like. 3–5 minutes.

This eye position affects the sixth chakra (energy centre) and strengthens the intuition.

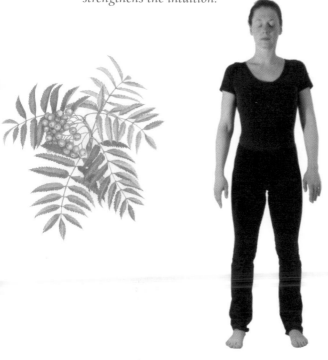

Relaxation
(standing, sitting or lying) 1–11 minutes
Listen to the whispering of the leaves, and the stillness that envelopes everything.

Meditation for new ideals

(YB 9 Jan. 1978)

Sit with your legs crossed and your spine straight. Put your right hand on the back of your left hand and hold both hands a couple of centimetres from, and just above, your heart centre. (This is the centre of your chest.) Let your elbows hang down.

Let your breath flow freely and just watch it. Your body will find its own breathing rhythm in this meditation.

Your eyes are 1/10 open and your gaze is on the tip of your nose. 11 minutes.

Use this meditation to acknowledge where your feelings come from. You will gain a feeling for your centre, your core, and will recognise your true ideals.

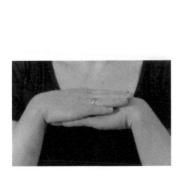
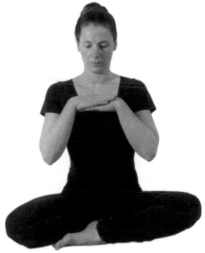

BEECH
(Fagus sylvatica)

We've all seen the hearts and messages carved into the patient, silver-grey trunks of beech trees. 'F.T. was here 18.3.1865', 'M loves S', and so on. The tree takes the message and retains it for hundreds of years. But the beech tree's association with the written word goes back much further than its being used for scrawling upon.

In all cultures, alphabets were originally created not as mere lists of phonetic symbols, but as systematic maps that express both the elemental forces of creation and the laws of nature. They were used by priests and shamans, principally for divination and prophecy. Much later in 'historical' times, new alphabets started to be used. Although they partially grew out of the ancient symbolic systems, individual symbols lost their meanings and only retained a phonetic function. Writing lost its solely religious dimension and started to be utilised to describe the contents of storerooms, for tax collection, and to record the great battles and conquests of powerful kings. This transition, then, marked the beginning of 'historical' time as compared to 'pre-history'. In pre-historical times the written word was magic: it retained the power of the spoken word by giving it duration through time. From the beginning, stone was used to facilitate this end; however, over time, lighter materials came into use. In Europe, for example, thin boards made from light-coloured beech wood were used. The Old High German word *buohhin*, 'from beech wood', became the word for 'book' in German and English. And the German word for 'letter', *Buchstabe*, literally means 'book stick' but also possibly 'beech stick', a reference to the divinatory runes that were carved on wooden sticks.

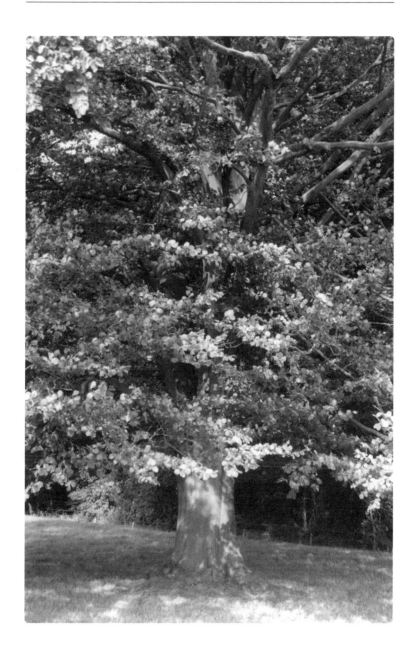

But even without the avid scribbling of humans, beech is the memory store of the woods. Naturally this is partially true of all trees, but more than any other species beech seems to retain the vibration of past events, whether they be battles, storms, or moments of beauty.

Interestingly, beech is also intimately connected with the planet Saturn, the astrological symbol of the force responsible for preservation, contraction, compression, and isolation. Trees that are connected to Saturn tend to create their own space: think of the dark stillness in spruce plantations; or of the sublime cathedral-like spaces within a beech wood, containing hardly a whisper of undergrowth, just the pure density of their unified energetic field. It is this compressing, concentrating quality that is responsible for changing leaves into needles, an excellent way of living in harsh climates. The beech obviously has leaves not needles, but its leaves are unusually small for a broad-leafed tree of such size and stature. Another difference is seen in the woody, slightly spiky seed casings of the beech, in contrast, for example, to its relation the oak and its exposed acorns.

At the same time as being connected to Saturn, beech is, like all broadleaved trees, ruled by the planet Jupiter. Jupiter is the force of expansion. Perhaps it is by embodying a balance of these two powers that the beech has become one of the most successful trees of the ancient forests of Western and Central Europe.

Beeches are full of vitality, and many people feel utterly invigorated just by walking among them. Their concentrated, condensed energies make them valuable and joyous companions. They can help us find clarity and inner purpose.

> The key words to attune to the spiritual qualities of the beech are *concentration, preservation, alignment* and *discipline.*

Exercise Sequence for Concentration

We recommend that you do these exercises underneath or in sight of a beech tree. If that isn't possible then visualise a beech tree. The energy of the tree strengthens the effect of the exercises.

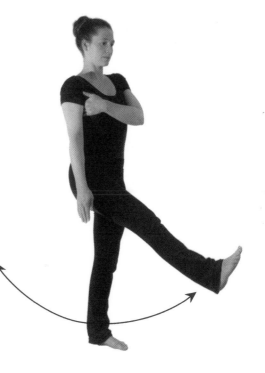

Concentration, Part 1

a) Stand upright and put your left hand under your right armpit. Your right arm hangs down straight by your side. As you breathe in, swing your left leg straight backwards, and breathe out as you swing it forwards. Sense that your swinging movement is coming from the middle of your body. Repeat this for 30 seconds, then change hand and leg before continuing for another 30 seconds.

This exercise brings spiritual clarity by stimulating the Nadis under the arm, which are connected to the brain. It also encourages the integration of the various body systems.

b) Stand upright and rotate your stretched-out arms backwards, making flowing circular movements. Your arms are following a straight line. As your right arm circles up, lift your right knee; and when your left arm is up, lift your left knee. Breathe long and deep, following the rhythm of the movement. 3 minutes.

This exercise harmonises the two hemispheres of the brain and gives alertness and clarity.

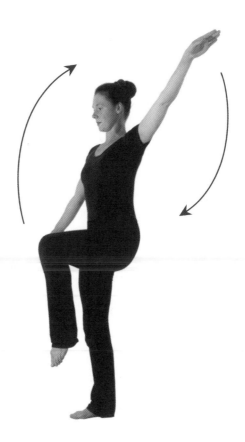

c) Stand upright with your feet together; bend your head forwards until your chin is touching the top of your chest, in-between your collar bones. Focus your attention on the upper part of your neck and do the Breath of Fire. 1–3 minutes. To finish, breathe in deeply and then gently bring your head level again to experience the after effects of the exercise.

This exercise works on the brain stem and the breath and sleep centres.

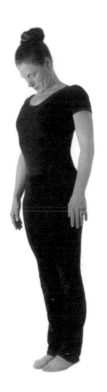

Concentration, Part 2

a) Place your feet hip-width apart. Stretch up your arms about 60 degrees apart, turn your palms so they face forwards, and spread your fingers far apart. In this pose breathe in deeply, and then as you breathe out cross your arms over your head and in front of you. Then spread your arms again as you breathe in. With the next breath, cross your arms the other way around, and so on. Keep your arms straight and make these movements quickly. Fix your gaze on a point on the tree trunk or a nearby wall. 4 minutes.

This exercise stimulates the meridians in the arms and teaches you to maintain your focus.

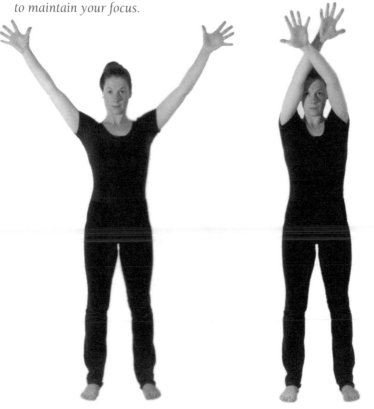

b) Place your arms hip-width apart and bend forwards from your hips. Support your hands on your hips, fingers pointing backwards, thumbs pointing forwards. Hold your head so that your neck follows a straight line from your back. Stretch your legs and stay in this position as you breathe long and deep. 1–3 minutes.

This exercise strengthens the main back muscles.

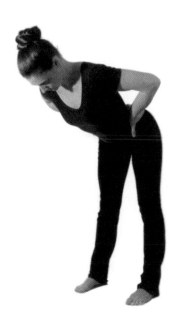

c) Stand upright with your feet together. Fix your gaze on a point on the ground about 1.5 meters from your toes. Breathe long and fully. 1–3 minutes.

This exercise strengthens the memory.

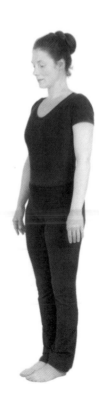

Concentration, Part 3

a) Place your feet hip-width apart, stretch up your arms and as you breathe in clap them over your head. As you breathe out clap them in front of your chest. Keep your arms stretched and eyes shut. 52 times.

This exercise activates the brain.

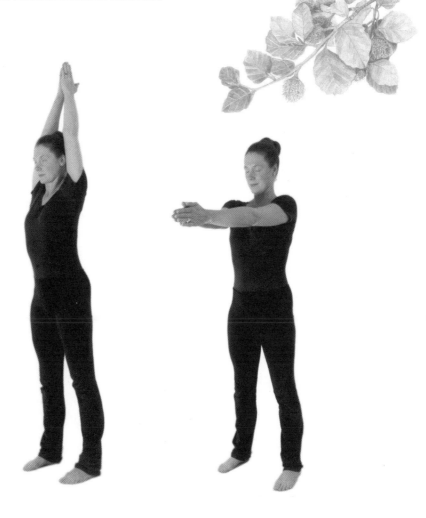

b) Breathe in and roll your eyes in large circles in one direction, breathe out and roll them in the other direction. 1–3 minutes.

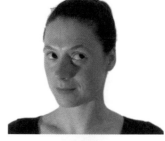

c) Look at an object and then move your eyes quickly around, each time coming back to look at the same object. Breathe long and slow. 1–3 minutes.

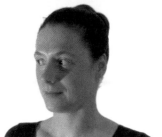

d) Move your eyes from looking top left to bottom right, and back again. After 10 times, change sides and look from bottom left to top right and back again. Breathe long and slow.

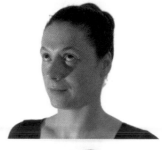

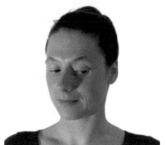

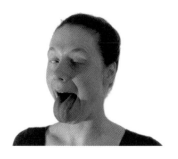

e) Stretch out your tongue and move your eyes in all directions. Breathe heavily through your mouth. 1–3 minutes.

The eye movements encourage the activity of the endocrine glands, while sticking out the tongue encourages spiritual clarity.

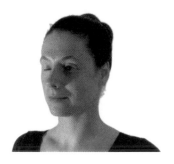

f) Shut one eye. Gently focus the other eye on an object. Breathe long and deep. 5 minutes per eye.

This exercise brings alignment and clarity.

Relaxation
(standing, sitting or lying) 1–11 minutes
Listen to the whispering of the leaves, and the stillness that surrounds everything.

Meditation for strong nerves
Sit cross legged, with your spine straight. Hold up your left hand so that it is level with your ear, palm forwards. At the same time touch the tip of your thumb and ring finger together. Lay your right hand in your lap, touching the tip of your thumb and little finger together. If you are a man, hold up your right hand instead and lay your left hand in your lap.

Keep your eyes about 1/10 open, look at the tip of your nose and breathe peacefully, long and deep.

To finish: breathe in deeply, open your fingers, lift up your hands and shake them vigorously for a minute or so as you breathe deeply. Then relax.

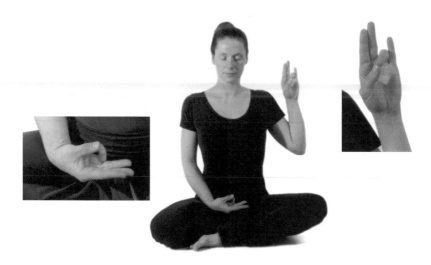

Start with 11 minutes per day and increase gradually over 30 days to 31 minutes.

The Mudra that brings together the ring finger, related to the sun, and the thumb, related to the self or 'I', instils new energy. The Mudra that brings together the thumb and little finger, related to the planet mercury, calms the nervous system and strengthens the ability to communicate.

PIPAL (BODHI)
(Ficus religiosa)

The pipal is the only non-Western tree in this book. Even though there are hardly any to be found in America or Europe that you could practice Yoga underneath (in Europe you'll generally only find a bodhi tree in a botanical garden), this wonderful being had to be included because of its great importance in Indian history and spirituality. *Tree Yoga* wouldn't be yoga without the pipal.

Together with the banyan *(Ficus bengalensis)* and the bel tree *(Aegle marmelos)*, the pipal has the longest history of tree worship in India. And 'history' really means something in this context because on the Indian subcontinent tree worship goes back over thousands of years. The earliest archaeological finds that record this are the Harappa seals (circa 2000 BC) and the image from Mohenjo-Daro (circa 3000 BC), but we can safely presume much earlier activity to have taken place. Also, as neither Hinduism nor Buddhism waged war on earlier nature religions in the way that Christianity has done throughout Europe and beyond, there are wonderfully complete records and handed-down teachings that include the worship of sacred trees. Examples are still to be found in some Indian village communities.*

Because of the scarcity of the pipal in Europe we have chosen exercises and meditations in this chapter that you can practice with any species of tree. Why? Because every tree can support us in the freeing of our spirit. You could look at this chapter as the joker in the pack, which can be used anywhere.

* The sacred trees of India are explored in greater depth in Fred's book *The Heritage of Trees*.

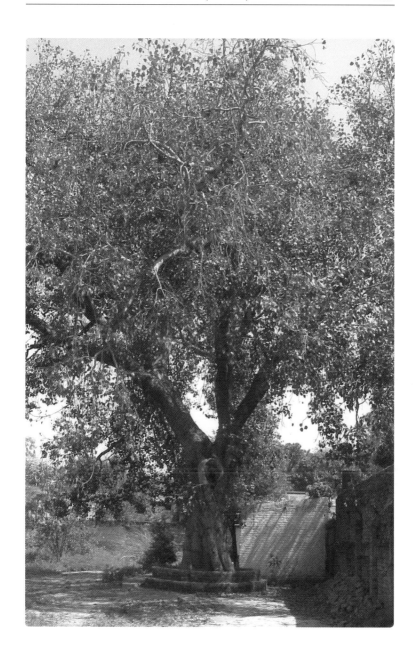

Since time immemorial the pipal has been a sacred tree. The *soma vessel* (*soma* is the life-giving sap of the World Tree) and the sacred fire stick were both fashioned from its wood. The Hindu trinity of Brahma, Vishnu and Shiva is portrayed as the three trunks of the World Tree. The very essence of Brahma is said to have materialised as the holy pipal tree. *Asvatha* is the religious name of the pipal and means 'that which won't be the same tomorrow.'

The *Bhagavad-Gita* describes the pipal as an incarnation of Krishna. At sacred tree shrines throughout India, the energies of Brahma, Krishna and the pipal are passionately celebrated.

About 2,500 years ago, the rich prince Gautama Siddhartha (circa 563–483 BC) rejected his material inheritance and position, and went off in search of spiritual freedom. Eventually he came to a powerful *Asvatha* tree shrine in northern India. After he had found enlightenment there, the pipal became known as the bodhi tree or Tree of Enlightenment, *bodhi* meaning 'ultimate and unconditioned truth', and also 'the Great Awakener'. During the first few hundred years of Buddhism, the Buddha was portrayed as an empty throne at the base of the Tree of Enlightenment, meaning that the person meditating at the base of the tree had overcome his human limitations and had become one with the spirit of the universe, the world spirit, the all-encompassing Tree of Life.

The key word to attune ourselves to the spirit of the pipal is *freedom.*

Exercise Sequence for Freedom

We recommend that you do these exercises underneath or in sight of a bodhi tree. If that isn't possible, then visualise a bodhi tree. The energy of the tree strengthens the effect of the exercises.

Freedom, Part 1

a) Place your feet hip-width apart; now alternate between standing on the balls of your feet and back down again. Keep your eyes shut. Firebreathe. 1–3 minutes.

The calf muscles are energetically connected to the lymph glands. These exercises stimulate the pituitary gland.

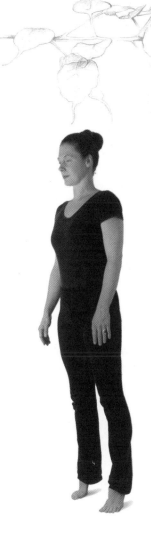

b) Stand on the balls of your feet. As you breathe in bring up your left knee, and then put it down again as you breathe out, coming back to your starting position. Now breathe in, lift your right knee, and then as you breathe out come back to the starting position again. Direct your gaze to a point on the bodhi tree or a nearby wall. 1–3 minutes per side.

This exercise also works on the pituitary gland; and on the inner ear, which is responsible for your balance.

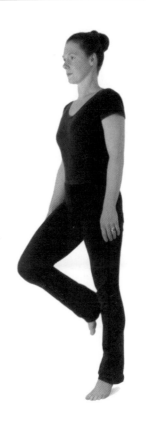

c) Crouching pose

Place your feet about 50 cm apart, and squat. Hold your arms in front of your chest, insides of your arms pointing forwards, and grasp your ankles. Lift your bottom until your back straightens. Stretch your tongue right out and firebreathe. 1.5–3 minutes.

This exercise is very cleansing. It also regulates the blood pressure in the brain.

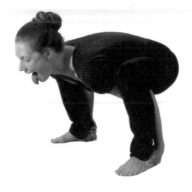

Freedom, Part 2

a) Place your feet hip-width apart. Clasp your fingers together and stretch out your forefingers together. Now stretch your arms high above your head, tighten your pelvic floor and bend forwards from the hips as you breathe out; and bend backwards, while still stretching your arms over your head, as you breathe in. 1–3 minutes.

This exercise works the calves and stimulates spiritual growth, (the forefinger represents Jupiter, which is symbolic of growth and wisdom.)

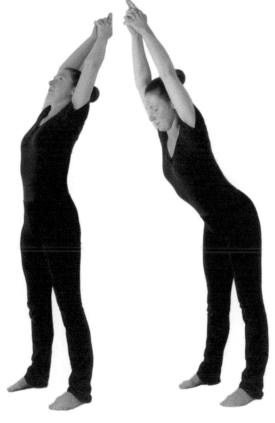

b) Place your feet about 50 cm apart and hold your arms parallel to the ground. Keep your eyes shut and your spine straight during this exercise. Breathe in and turn your upper body to the left, then breathe out and turn to the right. Your arms stay in one straight line. 3–5 minutes.

This exercise strengthens the heart and spine at the level of the chest.

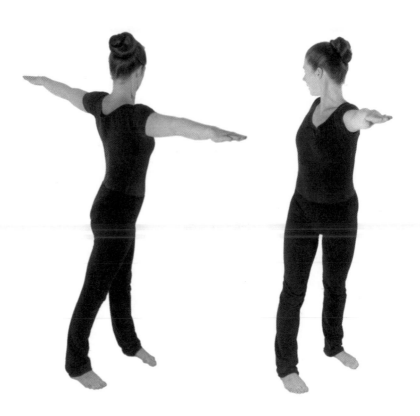

c) Place your feet hip-width apart. Clasp your fingers together and stretch out your forefingers together. Now stretch your arms high above your head, tighten your pelvic floor, shut your eyes and bend to your right, stretching your left hand side. Breathe long and deep. 1–3 minutes. Come back to the centre, breathe deeply, and then breathe out and bend to your left, stretching your right hand side. Breathe long and deep. 1–3 minutes.

This exercise stretches the sides of your body, particularly the intercostal muscles and large back muscles.

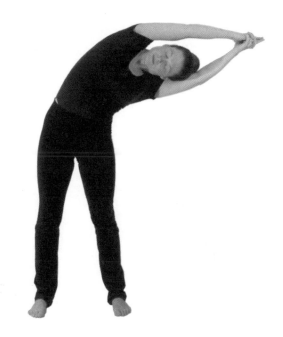

d) Place your feet about 50 cm apart and press them firmly into the ground. Stretch up your arms so that they are about 60 degrees apart, and hold your hands in the *Gyan Mudra*. As you breathe out bend your knees until your thighs are parallel to the ground, then stretch them up again as you breathe in. Your upper body stays upright. 3 minutes.

This exercise strengthens the heart and encourages the growth of new red blood cells.

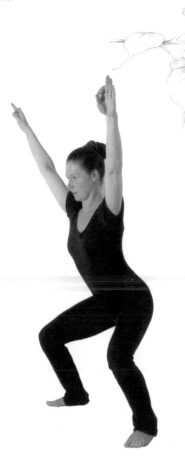

e) Place your feet about hip-width apart. Clasp your fingers together and stretch out your forefingers together. Now stretch your arms high above your head, and then make large circles with your upper body, moving from your hips. Breathe in as you go backwards and breathe out as you come forwards. Keep your eyes shut and focus your eyes on your third eye. 3 minutes, then change direction and 3 minutes more.

This exercise works the lumber and base of the spine, and hips. It frees spinal blocks.

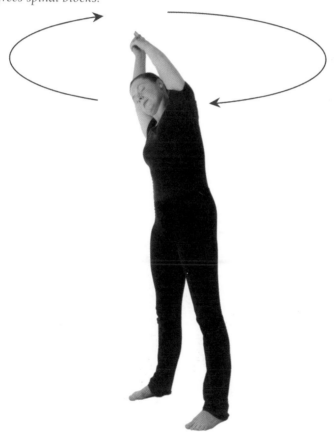

Freedom, Part 3

a) Placing your feet about hip-width apart, bend forwards while keeping your back straight and your head up. Stretch your arms out behind you and turn your palms downwards, spreading out your fingers. Direct your gaze to a point on the bodhi tree or a nearby wall. Breathe long and deep. 1–3 minutes.

This exercise strengthens the major back muscles, which are energetically connected to the spleen and pancreas meridian, and the so-called Life-Nadi (Nadi meaning energy current.)

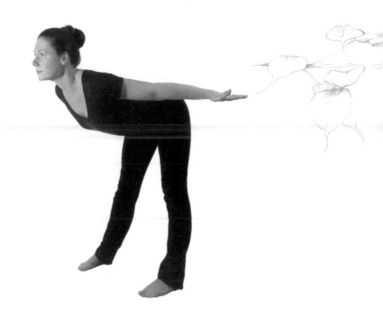

b) Stand upright and focus on your crown chakra. Roll up your eyes behind closed eyelids and imagine that you can see out of the crown of your head. Visualise a light at the top of your crown. Become conscious of the whole presence of the tree, above and below ground. Let the tree, or your imagined tree, help you in this. Breathe long and deep. 5 minutes.

This exercise increases your perceptive faculty, enabling you to sense atmospheres more clearly.

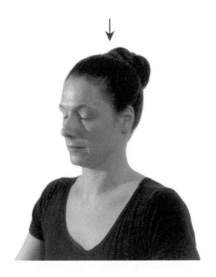

Relaxation
(standing, sitting, lying) 1–11 minutes.
Listen to the whispering of the leaves, and the stillness that surrounds everything.

Meditation for an expanded sense of self
(*YB 3 Feb. 1977*)
Sit with your legs crossed and your spine straight. Relax your hands in the middle of your lap. Shut your eyes and breathe peacefully and normally.

Imagine that you are sitting or standing on the top of a high mountain.

In your mind's eye, look down on the town or village where you live. Understand that what you can see down there is actually a part of you, and how expansive your mind and brain has to be to be able to contain all this.

Now imagine that you are travelling upwards until you can see the whole of the country where you live displayed before you, and that it too is a part of you.

Imagine that your perspective expands once more until you are looking at the whole of the earth, and can feel her inside of you. Understand that the whole of the planet is inside your head.

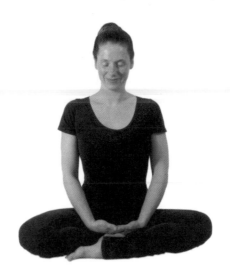

Stretch yourself even further and look at the whole of the solar system, then the whole of the universe. Continue to feel your body while simultaneously becoming the whole of the universe. Stretch out your small self, your 'I', so that it meets with your 'higher self'.

Go through the barriers of time and see if you can discover eternity. Stretch yourself out into the vast breadth and depth of your Self. In this expanse there is only pure light. It is a shimmering, simple, soft light.

Now imagine that this shimmering, simple, soft, beautiful, pure light is in the centre of your head. Turn your attention to it. Here is the pineal gland. It is the most precious jewel that God has given to you. Concentrate your whole self on this light. It is a blue light; it is subtle, warm and pure. It is inside your head, but is also as large as the entire cosmos.

Become pure light. Understand: 'I AM, I AM…!'

Give this your undivided attention and do it with great humility. As you perfect your ability to concentrate, your glands come into balance. Because of the effect on the endocrine glands, this meditation is particularly suited to the full moon, which is when the endocrine system shifts and becomes slightly imbalanced.

This meditation lets the inner light shine, and strengthens its radiation through and out of your body. For further guidance on this meditation, visit Satya's website: www.satyasingh.com/treeyoga

YEW
(Taxus baccata)

Both archaeology and mythology show that among Celtic and Germanic tribes the World Tree was above all celebrated in the form of the yew tree. Evidence of the remarkably pervasive spiritual importance of the yew goes back even further than this, far into the Stone Age, long before humanity formed itself into different cultural streams, back all the way in fact to the dawn of human consciousness. The yew grows in Europe and North America, and also throughout Asia. The oldest fossilised pieces of yew are 200 million years old, and the yew has not changed its genetic structure in the last 15 million years.

Some of the oldest and still living yew trees in Europe grow right next to Neolithic burial mounds (tumuli) that have been dated from 3000 BC to 1000 BC. These burial mounds were not just graves in the modern sense, they were places of magic, places where communities gathered to celebrate the seasonal festivals and make contact with the spirits of the ancestors. Yews often stand to the north of a tumulus – they are there as channels of energy and accompany the living as they make a leap in consciousness through the fabric of this world into the spirit world.

The yew is an example of one of the *few remaining unbroken lines* of European pre-Christian tradition: it has stayed connected to burial grounds through the Bronze Age, the Iron Age, the disquiet of mass migration, the Middle Ages and the epochs that have followed. Naturally yew trees and groves have also always existed outside of burial grounds, but almost all of these were sacrificed to the military's need for literally millions of longbows during the 15th and 16th centuries. Originally, for all cultures that rose within its natural distribution area, the yew was the tree of

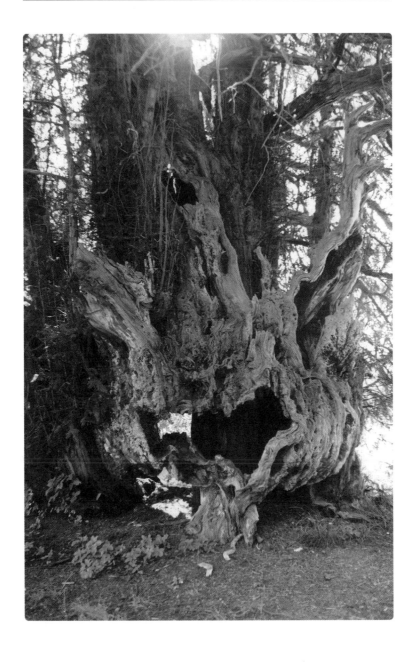

rebirth and eternity. This association is much deserved by this tree, which can grow into a peerless old age. Yews grow extremely slowly, which gives them a remarkable life span. Generally, unless they become fatally ill, trees die because they overtake themselves: at a certain point the biomass that is the crown becomes unmanageable for the transportation system that lies beneath the bark of the trunk and branches. Yews, however, are uniquely regenerative; at any moment in time, let's say after partial destruction of the crown, they can sprout new growth from anywhere beneath the bark. Yews can also grow trunks down to the ground where they can root themselves. In this way a single tree can transform itself into a circle of trees or even a grove. And sometimes so-called interior roots grow through the hollow trunk of an ancient yew and develop into a new trunk to support the crown. Thus the yew became a symbol of self-regeneration and rebirth. It is also an emblem of eternity because left to its own devices a yew can live for thousands of years.

In yew mythology we find references to immortality. The German rune *Eiwaz* signifies the yew tree and looks like a hook on which one might hang a cauldron or cooking pot over an open fire. The cauldron is another symbol of rebirth, and in Celtic tradition is also the vessel in which the consciousness-expanding drink known as the 'poet's mead' is brewed. This drink promises omniscience (compare *soma*, the sap from the Tree of Life). The yew is the agent, we could say *gate-keeper*, who stands between the worlds.

Some sources give the crushed bark of the yew tree as the substance once used to make the red mark known as the *bindhi* that is commonly painted throughout India on the third eye (in the middle of the forehead). It is also indicated that the *Brahmans* once used the toxic yew alkaloids to make *soma*. The sacred status of the Himalayan yew *(Taxus wallichiana)* appears to have been lost over time. Its old name, *deodaru*, 'tree of God', was eventually given to the Himalayan cedar *(Cedrus deodara)*.

> The key words to attune yourself to the spirit of the yew are *rebirth*, *destiny*, *timelessness* and *eternity*.

Exercise Sequence for Vitality

We recommend that you do these exercises underneath or in sight of a yew tree. If that isn't possible then visualise a yew tree. The energy of the tree strengthens the effect of the exercises.

Vitality, Part 1

a) Stand upright; stretch out your arms level in front of you and hold them firmly all the way into the tips of your fingers, so that they bend upwards a little. Close your eyes and breathe long and deep. 5 minutes.

This exercise energises the fingers, which reflexology teaches us are energetically connected to the brain and sinuses.

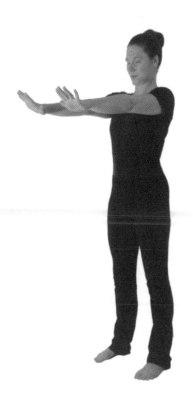

b) Stand upright, and again stretch your arms out level in front of you; hold them stiffly and breathe in. As you then breathe out, bend forwards from your hips while pulling up your pelvic floor, keeping your back straight, until your hands come down towards the ground, then relax your arms. As you breathe in, stand up again. Repeat for 5 minutes.

Relaxes the arms and strengthens the aura.

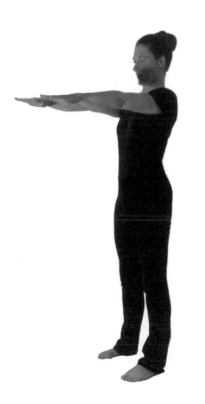
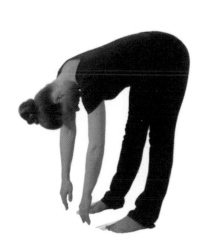

c) Stand upright and hold your elbows at shoulder height; bring your forearms in towards your chest and let your hands hang down. Now strongly tense your arms while keeping your hands relaxed. The Breath of Fire. 1–3 minutes.

This exercise relaxes the nervous system.

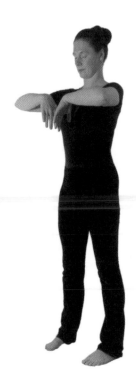

d) Stand upright and hold out your arms in front of you, parallel to the ground. Keep your fingers straight and palms facing forwards, now bend your wrists up and down quickly so that as you breathe in you are bending them as far up as they will go, and as you breathe out as far down as they will go. 1–3 minutes.

This exercise stimulates the meridians that run along the under-arms and strengthens the healing power of the hands.

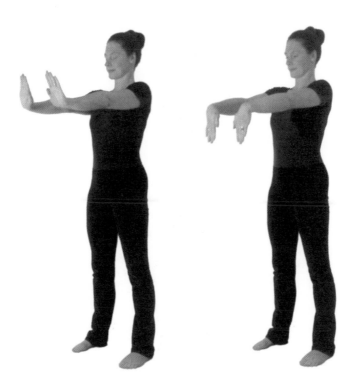

Vitality, Part 2

a) Stand upright and jump as high as you can ten times. Breathe in as you jump up and out as you land.

This exercise works the musculature of the calves, which are energetically connected to the lymphatic system, and increases the circulation.

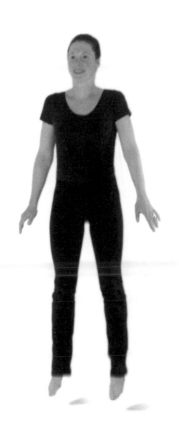

b) Place your feet hip-width apart. Stretch your arms out to the front, parallel to the ground, and make a fist with both hands. Breathe in and bend your fists up as far as they will go, then breathe out and bend them as far down as they will go. 1–3 minutes.

This exercise strengthens the wrists and underarms, and so also the triple heater (lymph) meridian.

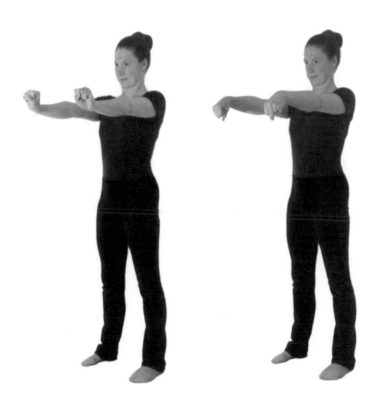

Vitality, Part 3

a) Place your feet hip-width apart and stretch your arms to the side at a 60-degree angle. Turn your palms forwards and spread out your fingers. Move your hands sideways, bending them from the wrists, and then quickly move them up and down. Shut your eyes and let your breath flow freely.

This exercise strengthens the nervous system. The 60-degree angle guides the energy into your heart.

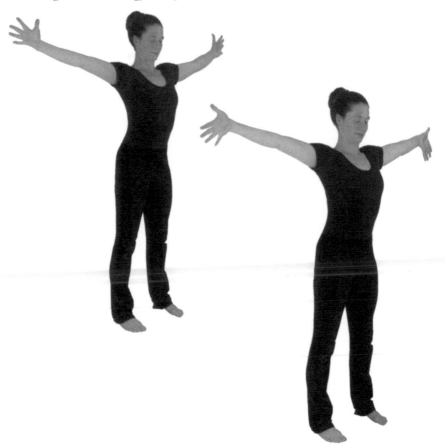

b) Stand upright and shut your eyes. Direct your eyes to your third eye. Breathe long and deep. 5 minutes.

The eye muscles stimulate the pituitary gland, which governs our intuition and insight.

Relaxation
(standing, sitting, lying) 1–11 minutes.
Listen to the quiet hum of life in the crown of the tree, and the stillness that envelops everything.

Bandha Dhya Kriya

(YB 27 October 1975)

Find a comfortable position in which to meditate.

Hold your hands about 15 cm in front of your heart centre, and gently press the outside edges of your hands together so that your little fingers (Mercury) are also touching each other. Now bend both your middle fingers (Saturn) until the ends touch one another and they stand at a 90-degree angle to your palms. Take care that your ring fingers (Sun) don't come into contact with each other.

Breathe in through your nose, filling your lungs in eight equal steps. Breathe out by whistling. Make sure you fully empty your lungs.

Don't practice this meditation for more than 11 minutes at first. With regular practice for one week, add a minute per week to build up to 31 minutes.

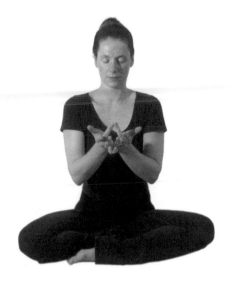

In the words of Yogi Bhajan:

'Carry out this Kriya with deep respect, love and dedication in a very peaceful way. Anything that is about Prana should be treated with the utmost respect, because Prana is the container of life.

This Kriya was kept very secret and only recommended to a chosen few. Tell a friend if you want to practice it. If the energy becomes too strong this person should wipe your face with a wet hand towel and give you a glass of water to drink. Don't practice this Kriya for more than 11 minutes until you have become accustomed to its power.

Bandha Kriya is very healing for the psyche. By practicing it you will be able to rise beyond the confines of time and space. After you have practiced it your problems will appear to be far smaller than they usually are. This is a beautiful and powerful meditation. Be quiet and humble with it. All will be well.'

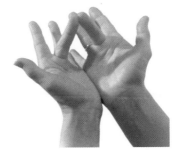

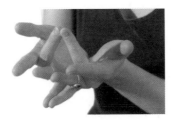

OAK
(Quercus)

If there is one species of tree that everybody knows (if not the birch), it is the oak. The oak deserves its fame for the way that it has helped to build and maintain human civilisation. Its wood has served for buildings, tools, doors and furniture, and also for making battleships for the imperialistic navies. During the Middle Ages an important part of the economy was the rearing of pigs, and every autumn hordes of pigs were driven into the rich oak and beech woodland to be fattened up. Also, the passing of the Dark Ages into the relative security of the Middle Ages would hardly have been possible without the 'economic aid' of the oak tree.

Of course it hasn't been just during historical time that the oak has been a blessing for humankind. It has played its role far longer than that. The Celts loved to hunt in oak forests, as did the Anglo-Saxons, and the warriors of both prized its wood for making battlements. But despite, or perhaps because of, the extent of its connections to masculine activities such as warfare and hunting, the oak is a rather 'maternal', nurturing tree. It is home and nourishment for over 500 types of insects, spiders, birds and other animals, which is far more than any other tree species in the temperate zone.

For the ancients, the oak was dedicated to the gods of sky and thunder: in Scandinavia, Thor; for the Celts, Taranis; and for the Greeks, Zeus. And indeed, oaks are struck by lightening more often than any other tree. It is assumed that this is because oaks often grow directly over underground watercourses or waterways. But their extraordinarily high level of electrical activity could also play a role.

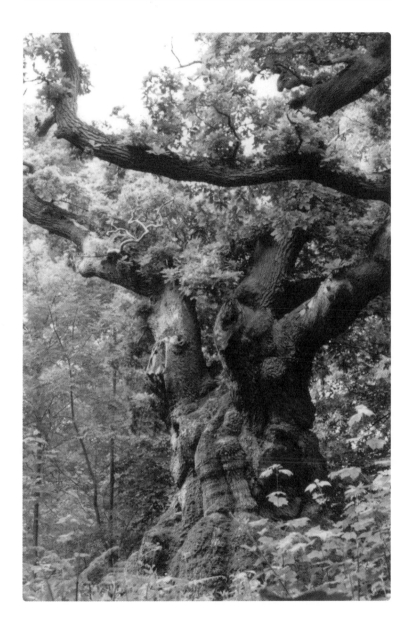

The Celtic name for the oak is related to the word for *door* (from the Sanskrit *dur*). This association exists because oaks can be used as doors to other planes of consciousness, and it is for this reason that they can be discovered in the sacred temples of some of the ancients. The clearest example of this is the connection between the oak and the Greek-Hellenic sky-god Zeus, whose name means 'the shining or bright one'. His well-known capacity for firing lightening bolts symbolises the incomparable power and dynamism with which his divine consciousness can manifest itself on earth. The symbolism of Zeus' lightening bolt has a direct parallel in certain Tibetan ritual objects *(dorjes)*, the religious significance of both being related to the expansion of consciousness.

All trees absorb and work with not just water, air and minerals, but also with frequencies, radiation sources, and pure information that originate both from the earth and from the cosmos. So every tree has a unique character and special resonance, which causes something in our soul to resonate too, stimulating different states of being and the life skills that go with them. The oak tree is a unique case in this respect because it doesn't display specific qualities but rather just pure life energy. The first thing we discover is that this extraordinary force is neutral and people can and have used it to fulfil their desires whether they be war or peace, healing, poetry, making important decisions, or for tree-yoga and raising their Kundalini. The spirit of the oak supports our earth journey, but not through the birthing phase like the birch, but through the stages of maturity and ripening.

> The key words that attune us to the energy of the oak are *life energy*, *strength* and *determination*.

Exercise Sequence for Willpower

We recommend doing these exercises under or in view of an oak tree. If that isn't possible, visualise an oak tree. The energy of the tree strengthens the positive effect of the exercise.

Willpower, Part 1

a) Place your feet hip-width apart. Quickly turn your head from left to right as if you were shaking your head. Keep your eyes shut and turn your eyes to your third eye, between your eyebrows. Breathe long and deep. 1 minute. Then quickly raise and lower your head as if you were nodding. You are stretching your throat and neck. Focus and breathe as before. 1 minute.

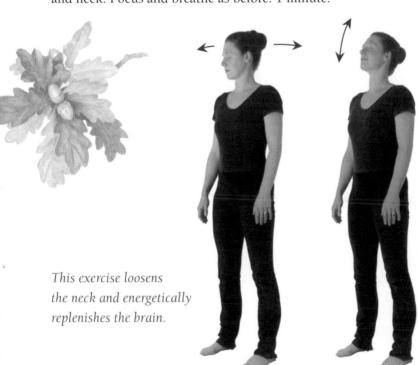

This exercise loosens the neck and energetically replenishes the brain.

b) Weightless running. Support your hands on the tree trunk, on a knee- or hip-high stool, or a windowsill. Run on the spot, kicking your heels into your bottom muscles as you run. Breathe long and deep. 3–10 minutes.

This exercise improves the circulation in the legs.

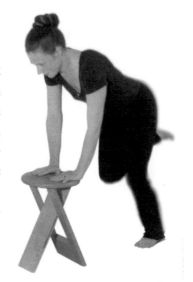

c) Place your feet 50 cm apart. As you breathe in, swing your left arm straight over your body to your right thigh without moving the rest of your body.
At
the same
time, holding your right arm at a 45-degree angle, swing it backwards. Repeat these movements in the opposite direction. Keep your eyes shut, and direct them to your third eye. 3 minutes.

This exercise integrates the right and left sides of the body.

Willpower, Part 2

a) Place your feet about 65 degrees apart and put your hands on your thighs. Breathe in, stretch your legs, and keep your upper body horizontal. Lift your head away from your shoulders and stretch your throat. Maintaining the same position with your upper body, straighten your knees as you breathe out. As you breathe in, bend them again. Keep your back straight. Repeat in rhythm with your breath. 2 minutes.

This exercise strengthens the thighs.

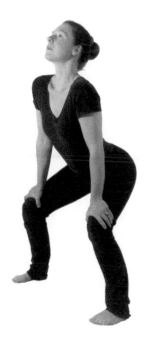
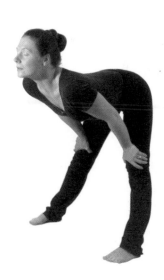

b) Place your feet hip-width apart; bend to the front with straight legs and put your hands around your calves. (If you have back problems put your hands on your knees or thighs.) Breathe in and lift your head away from your shoulders, and bend your spine downwards so that it resembles the bowed back of a cow, while raising your bottom up. Breathe out and bring your chin down to your chest, round your back like a cat, and pull in your stomach. Keep your eyes shut. 3–7 minutes.

This exercise tones the back and increases flexibility.

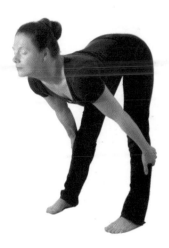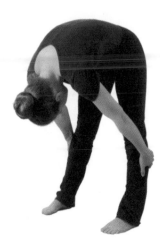

c) Place your feet hip-width apart and put your hands on your shoulders with your fingers pointing forwards and your thumbs backwards. Lift and hold your pelvic floor muscles. As you breathe in, stretch backwards at a 30-degree angle from your hips. As you breathe out, do the same forwards. Keep your eyes shut. 2 minutes.

This exercise cleanses the nerves and liver.

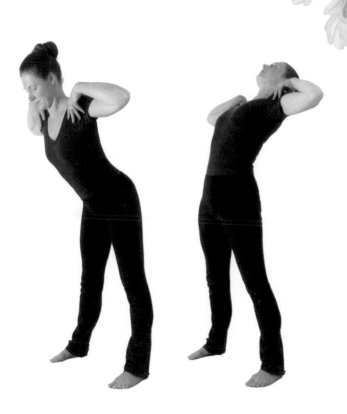

d) Place your feet hip-width apart; place your hands on your shoulders with your fingers facing forwards and your thumbs backwards. As you breathe in, turn your upper body and head to the left; as you breathe out turn them to the right. Shut your eyes and direct them to your third eye, between your eyebrows. Keep your spine straight. 2 minutes.

This exercise is both centring and increases the coordination between the two hemispheres of the brain.

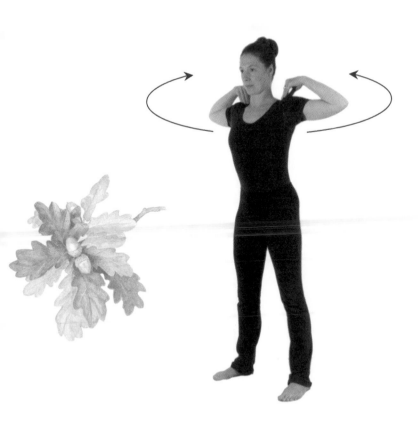

Willpower, Part 3

a) Place your feet hip-width apart; make a fist with both hands and swing your outstretched arms forwards in large circles. Shut your eyes and breathe long and deep. 1–3 minutes.

This exercise cleanses the aura and coordinates the five brain centres.

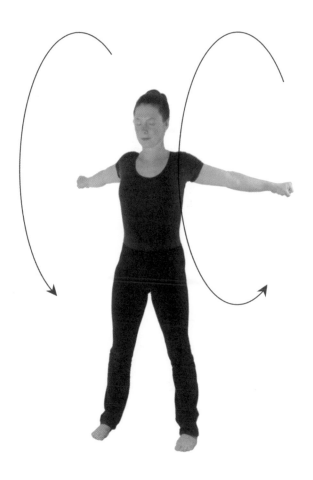

b) Place your feet about 60 cm apart; bend your upper body forwards and hold it horizontal to the ground. Lift your head away from your shoulders as if looking far into the distance. Shut your eyes and turn them to your third eye. Stretch your arms behind you, holding them up high and spreading your fingers apart. In quick succession, open and close your hands. Breathe long and deep. 3 minutes.

This exercise increases determination.

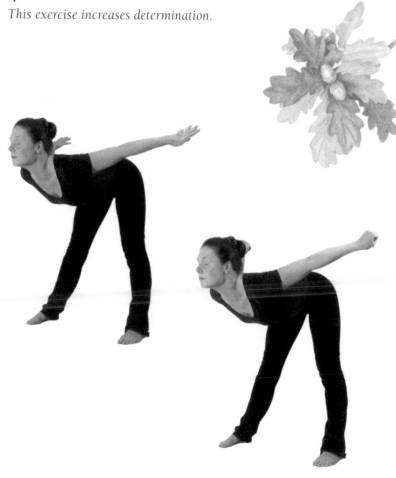

c) Bring your feet together so they are touching; extend your neck and bring up your chin until your throat is stretched as far as it will go. Keep your mouth shut, and open your eyes wide. The Breath of Fire. 1–3 minutes. To end with, breathe in deeply and gently and bring your head back to the vertical.

This exercise improves the memory.

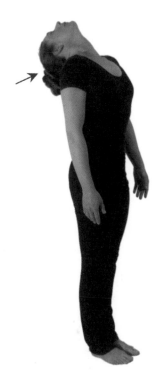

Relaxation
(standing, sitting or lying down) 1–11 minutes
Listen to the whispering of the leaves, and the stillness that surrounds everything.

Breath of Ten

(YB 8 May 1995)

Sit with your legs crossed and your back straight. Hold your hands in front of your chest, with your palms facing each other. Move your hands slowly and rhythmically as if you were clapping, but without touching. Stop when your hands are about 15 cm apart.

Breathe in through your nose in 5 graduated steps, and out through your mouth also in five graduated steps. With every one of the five intakes of breath, move your hands close to one another in one movement. Breathe and move your arms in a unified rhythm. Concentrate on the energy that you may feel between your hands. 11 minutes.

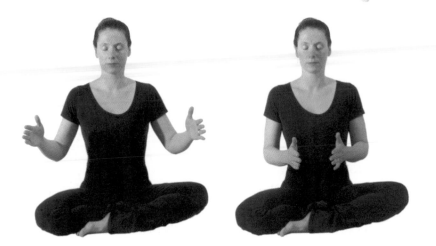

To end with breathe in, hold your breath, and strongly press your hands against your face for twenty seconds. Breathe out. Breathe in again, hold your breath, and press your hands to your heart for twenty seconds. Breathe out. Breathe in and press your hands to your navel for twenty seconds. Breathe out and take it easy.

This exercise is therapeutic for your electromagnetic field. While doing it, the energetic connection between your hands should be continuous. The Breath of Ten is a complete breath similar to the Breath of Fire. This exercise stimulates the regulatory system in your brain that controls your immune system. If you practice this meditation for 11 minutes a day, all of your chakras will be brought into a health-giving pattern. This will leave your body healthy and your spirit clear; a sense of energised peace comes about and your intuition is awakened.

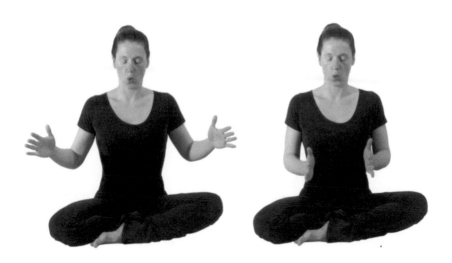

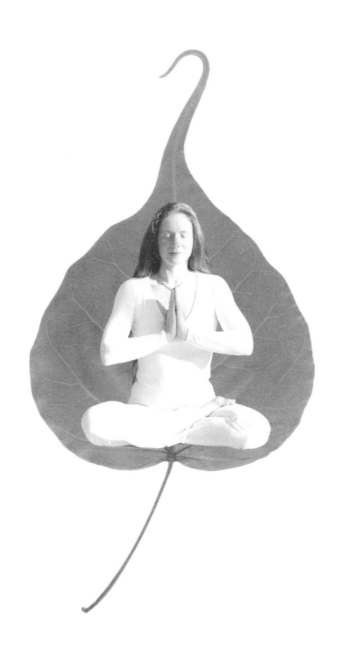

The Authors

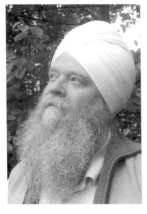 **Satya Singh** was born in 1949 in Haarlem, the Netherlands. In 1974 he started studying as a personal student of Yogi Bhajan, which he remained until Yogi Bhajan's parting from this world in 2004. He has lived in Ashrams in Amsterdam and Hamburg, and continued his studies with yearly visits to the USA, France and India. Satya has written two books in German. In 1990 his *Kundalini Yoga handbook for the health of body, mind and soul* was published, and has since become a standard text for Kundalini Yoga. Meeting with continuous enthusiasm from readers, the book has been translated into four languages. In 2000, *The Ring*, a Yoga novel, was published. This is a gripping story of personal discovery through Yoga, set in Cyprus and the Himalayas.

He sees his work as passing on the inner light and healing that he has gained through the systematic practice of Kundalini Yoga. The most effective way of doing this is to educate students to become teachers of Kundalini Yoga, as Yogi Bhajan instructed, 'If you want to know something read about it, if you want to learn something, study it, if you want to master something, teach it!' Satya leads a team of Kundalini Yoga instructors who teach teachers in ten German cities and a number of European Countries.

Satya's vision and hope for Tree Yoga is that we learn to prize nature not just for its beauty and usefulness, but also as partner, helper and healer on our personal spiritual path.

Satya is a member of 3HO International, which promotes Yogi Bhajan's teachings worldwide. For info go to:
www.3ho.org or www.satyasingh.com

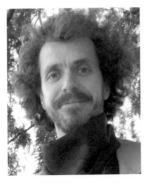 **Fred Hageneder**, born in 1962 in Hamburg, Germany, is an author, musician, graphic designer and lecturer, who has studied trees passionately since 1980, in conjunction with comparative religion, cultural history, mythology and archaeology. Fred has become a leading author in ethnobotany and the cultural and spiritual history and meaning of trees. So far, his work has been translated into German, Dutch, Spanish, Italian, Esthonian, Polish and Czech. He has given lectures in various ecology centres in Britain, Germany and Switzerland, and at the Abant Izzet Baysal University in Turkey. His publications include *The Spirit of Trees* (2000) and *The Heritage of Trees* (2001), two companion volumes exploring the cultural relationships of humanity and trees in the past, and *The Living Wisdom of Trees*, a study of past and present living tree culture and myths worldwide (2005). *Yew – A History* (2007) is his fourth book on the cultural history of trees.

Fred is a member of the AYG (Ancient Yew Group, www.ancient-yew.org), an independent research group, and co-founder of Friends of the Trees (www.FriendsOfTheTrees.org.uk), a registered charity that aims to promote modern tree sanctuaries as oases of peace, as well as cross-cultural and inter-faith meeting places.

Previously published works include:

The Spirit of Trees: Science, Symbiosis and Inspiration. Floris Books, Edinburgh 2000

The Heritage of Trees: History, Culture and Symbolism. Floris Books, Edinburgh 2001

The Living Wisdom of Trees: Natural History, Folklore, Symbolism, Healing. Duncan Baird Publishers, London 2005

Yew – A History. Sutton Publishing, Stroud 2007

Recommended Literature

Yoga for Skiers and Runners. Nirvair Singh Khalsa, 1994

Kundalini Yoga/Sadhana Guidelines. Yogi Bhajan. Kundalini Research Institute 1974

Kundalini Yoga. Shakta Kaur Khalsa. DK 2001

The Teachings of Yogi Bhajan. Hawthorne Books 1977

Kundalini, the Essence of Yoga. Guru Dharam Singh Khalsa & Darryl O'Keefe. Gaia Books 2002

Keeping up with Kundalini Yoga. Yogi Bhajan. Kundalini Research Institute 1980

Yoga for the 80's. Yogi Bhajan. Arcline Institute 1982

Kundalini Yoga Manual, Student Manual of Instruction. Yogi Bhajan. Kundalini Research Institute 1976

Kundalini Yoga Maintenance Manual. Yogi Bhajan. Kundalini Research Institute 1977

Self Experience. Yogi Bhajan. Kundalini Research Institute 2000

Energy Maps, a Journey through the Chakras. Guru Darshan Kaur. Cyber Scribe 1991

Sexuality and Spirituality. Yogi Bhajan by Guru Rattan Kaur, 1989

Introduction to Kundalini Yoga. Gururattan Kaur & Ann Marie Maxwell, 1989

Transitions to a Heart Centered World. Gururattan Kaur & Ann Marie Maxwell, 1988

Reaching Me in Me, Kundalini Yoga as taught by Yogi Bhajan. Kundalini Research Institute, 2002

Relax and Renew, with the Kundalini Yoga and Meditations of Yogi Bhajan. Gururattan Kaur Khalsa, 1988

Self Knowledge, Kundalini Yoga as taught by Yogi Bhajan. Yogi Bhajan, 1995

Owners Manual for the Human Body, Kundalini Yoga as taught by Yogi Bhajan. KIT 1993

Physical Wisdom, Kundalini Yoga as taught by Yogi Bhajan. Ancient Healing Ways 1994

Infinity and Me, Kundalini Yoga as taught by Yogi Bhajan. Kundalini Research Institute 2004

Divine Alignment. Guruprem Singh Khalsa, 2003

Some of the above are available through your bookshop or at:
www.satnam.de   www.a-healing.com

Other interesting websites:
www.satyasingh.com   www.3ho.org
www.kriteachings.org   www.kundaliniyoga.com
www.spirit-of-trees.de   www.ancient-yew.org
www.friendsofthetrees.org.uk

Picture Credits

Cover photo of Satnam Kaur Wester by Satya Singh.

All yoga poses taken by Satya Singh and Fred Hageneder;
    model: Avtar Kaur Olivier.

All tree photos taken by Fred Hageneder, apart from rowan and
    oak, taken by Simant Bostock, and the pipal, taken by Satya
    Singh.

All tree illustrations: Elaine Vijaya

Illustrations:

1, 2, 3 from *The Spirit of Trees*

4, Elaine Vijaya from *The Spirit of Trees*

5, from A.B. Cook, *Zeus*, 1914, pp. 229 and 402

Photo of Yogi Bhajan, p. 33: unknown

Illustrations, p. 46–47 Angela Schneider

Photos p. 215: Fred Hageneder

Photo p. 216: Gisela Winnnig

Photo p. 217: Elaine Vijaya

Afterword

In his usual modesty, Yogi Bhajan described himself as nothing more than a messenger:

'I don't take anything away, I don't add anything; I just pass on the gifts that have been given to me.'

Out of thanks for his remarkable message, the authors are donating 10% of their proceeds from this book to the international institutions that make Yogi Bhajan's teachings accessible to the general public.

May the long time sun
shine upon you
All love surround you
And the pure light within you
Guide your way on

Sat Nam

Bringing Together Human and Tree

What is a 'sacred' grove?
In the ancient cultures of Classical Greece, Rome and Egypt, as well as the woodland tribes of the Celts or Anglo-Saxons there were trees of a sacred status that were protected from harm and were respected by people who had a deeper understanding of nature. These were places of celebration and joy, not feared. Sometimes gifts or offerings (flowers, fruits, candles, ribbons tied to the branches) were left there to express gratitude to the Source of all Life. These were natural temples, places with a powerful and peaceful atmosphere. One doesn't have to be religious to sense this. We would experience it as a special place. Such places still exist in India and Japan today.

A sacred grove is a special place but without the architecture of a cathedral or temple. And without this historical and cultural context it is equally welcoming to a Hindu, a Buddhist, a Moslem, a Christian or a Jew. All of these religions have sacred trees in their own traditions.

The Friends of the Trees hope to create special places of contemplation, peace, and mutual friendship in nature.

• Peaceful and quiet places where you can feel at ease with yourself and your environment.
• Places that teach us something about true ecology and where we find our power to give back to nature, in our own special ways.
• Places as environmental care in action, which make it tangible and joyful!
• Places where we can find inspiration, relaxation and healing.
• Places that might awaken us to something more within ourselves.

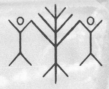

Friends of the Trees

Friends of the Trees
The Secretary · 269 Melbourne Court · Battlefield ·
Newcastle on Tyne · NE1 2AU · www.FriendsOfTheTrees.org.uk

There are two types of angels: those with wings, and those with leaves. For thousands of years, those seeking advice or wanting to give thanks to Mother Nature have walked the ancient paths into the sacred grove. Because today sacred groves have become scarcer, and venerable old trees in tranquil spots are hard to find

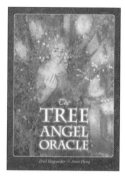

when we need them, Earthdancer is pleased to present this tree oracle to bring the tree angels closer to us all once more.

Fred Hageneder, Anne Heng
The Tree Angel Oracle
36 colour cards (95 x 133 mm)
plus book, 112 pages
ISBN 978-1-84409-078-5

Beautiful music inspired by our native trees, performed on harp, flute, strings and various surprises. Rooted in a deep understanding of trees and their myths and history, this album is dedicated to ten tree species that have been of outstanding importance in the spiritual history of western Europe since the earliest times.

A musical mystical journey, both meditative and rhythmic, full of colour, change and movement, yet breathing a deep tranquillity.

Fred Hageneder
The Spirit of Trees
CD, 66 min.
Music for harp, flute, strings and more.

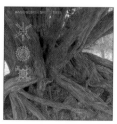

For further information and book catalogue contact:
Findhorn Press, 305a The Park, Forres IV36 3TE, Scotland.
Earthdancer Books is an Imprint of Findhorn Press.

tel +44 (0)1309-690582   fax +44 (0)1309-690036
info@findhornpress.com
www.earthdancer.co.uk   www.findhornpress.com

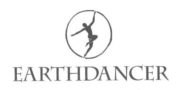

A FINDHORN PRESS IMPRINT